A Basic Guide to Growing Herbs

A Basic Guide to Growing Herbs

With an Introduction to Healing Herbs

Fee O'Shea

© 2019 by Fee O'Shea

All Rights Reserved.
No part of this publication may be reproduced in any form or by any means, including scanning, photocopying, or otherwise without prior written permission of the copyright holder.

Terms of Use

You are given a non-transferable, "personal use" license to this product. You cannot distribute it or share it with other individuals.

Also, there are no resale rights or private label rights granted when purchasing this document. In other words, it's for your own personal use only.

Printed in: USA
First published: 2019
ISBN: 978-0-473-48006-6

- INTRODUCTION 7
  - HOW TO USE THIS BOOK WISELY. 8
- CHAPTER ONE: WHY HERBS? 13
  - CULINARY HERBS. 14
  - AROMATIC HERBS. 17
  - ORNAMENTAL HERBS. 17
  - MEDICINAL HERBS. 19
  - THE ANCIENT CHINESE KNEW THEIR HERBS! 20
  - MANY A PRESCRIPTION DRUG DERIVED FROM HERBS. 22
  - TEA TIME! 24
- CHAPTER TWO: WHICH HERBS? 27
  - TOP 10 CULINARY HERBS. 28
  - GROWING MEDICINAL HERBS? TOP TEN HEALING HERBS. 36
- CHAPTER THREE: DESIGN A GARDEN 53
- CHAPTER FOUR: OUTDOOR GARDENING 73
- CHAPTER FIVE: INDOOR GARDENING 85
- CHAPTER SIX: CARING FOR THE HERBS. 97
- CHAPTER SEVEN: PREPARING HERBAL REMEDIES. 111
- CHAPTER EIGHT: 14 TIPS TO HELP YOU GET STARTED 119
- CONCLUSION. 123
- APPENDIX I: WHAT YOUR HERBS NEED. 125
  - ANNUAL HERBS. 125
  - BIENNIAL AND PERENNIAL HERBS. 128
- REFERENCES 138

Introduction

Is it the influence of the "Green Movement?" Or is it the growing concern over the economy? Or perhaps it's just the love of herbs have finally gotten hold of enough people to create the interest in herb gardening we see today.

Whatever the reason you may have for wanting to grow your own herbs, be it for your health, to put into your food or just because they are beautiful - Congratulations!

Once you begin you will wake up every day, walk out onto your patio or terrace or into your backyard and you will thoroughly enjoy the fragrance and visual beauty that will greet you.

Now you will have the opportunity to create culinary masterpieces, improve not only your health but those you are close to as well or just enrich your life.

Herbs really are easy to grow so long as you provide them with the conditions that they like, most of them will actually take the least amount of care in your garden.

Because herbs are so easy to grow, if you're a beginning gardener, then they are an absolute must. Embracing herbs will give you the confidence you need to go on to more difficult plants.

If, on the other hand, you are a really experienced gardener, then you will certainly appreciate these amazing plants for that very same reason. Once you have created your garden, it doesn't take much on your part to get it to look absolutely spectacular and keep it that way. (And, take all the credit your guests will toss your way!)

Of course, it goes without saying that you can just add dabs of colours and textures to an otherwise dreary patch of your flower garden. There are many gardeners who use herbs to separate flowers whose colours may clash or place them where no flower would succeed in growing.

If you have a damp, shady spot in your garden where nothing else grows, try an herb. As you delve deeper into this hobby, you'll learn how easy ... and common this can be.

Or perhaps you're just interested in planting a few herbs in a couple of containers to begin with. Another alternative is to keep several herbs potted on your back porch. Or even just grow only a very few of these culinary plants.

How to use this book wisely.

This book is designed to help you learn more about the wonderful plants you're about to adopt.

Chapter one answers the question that's on everyone's mind (while maybe not everyone's ...but probably yours): Why

Herbs? In this chapter we ask the questions about why you're drawn to growing herbs. What your answers reveal will be not only the type of garden you'll probably end up planting, but the various kinds of herbs you'll probably include in it.

Chapter two digs a little deeper (pardon the pun) on the subject of herbs. Once you've taken the step to examine why you want to grow herbs, then you can intelligently decide exactly which herbs you want to grow.

Now granted your first year of gardening might be a bit of a hit and miss. Don't worry, if you're truly successful at gardening, it will be. You won't really want to stop once you start learning about herbs. By the end of your first growing season, you'll have a list of extra herbs you will want to include in your next venture. Which will be brilliant!

Also in this chapter you will find some of the most popular herbs used in both culinary practice and also for healing. It won't take long to discover that it's nigh on impossible to give them a strict classification.

For example let's take Basil. Most people typically think that basil is used only for culinary delights; however, this gorgeous herb also works as an anti-inflammatory remedy. So if you do decide to grow basil for the kitchen, you just could end up using it for your health as well!

Now in Chapter Three, we look at the design of the garden. This will help you to decide what type of garden you want as well as how to bring it to life. We will explore all the options and figure out what is going to work best for your lifestyle as well as your culinary and health needs.

In Chapter Four, I've got you covered if you have decided to have an outdoor garden. Things like how to grow the herbs in your own backyard as well as hints, tips and suggestions. This is a great chapter to get a good jumpstart to your herb hobby.

Perhaps you'd prefer to begin with an indoor garden? Then you'll need to read up on Chapter Five because this will make sure that your herbal expedition indoors is very successful.

Now, onto Chapter Six, which is a general overview of the best ways to keep your herbs healthy, happy and strong. This chapter will reassure you that you certainly can maintain an herb garden, so it will dispel any doubts you may have.

Right at the end in Chapter Seven I give you fifteen tips, some of which are a re-cap of what I've written. These tips are there to help you get it clear in your mind just what to keep a look out for once you have decided where you are going to plant and which herbs you will pick. And I tell you who your best friend is!

A Basic Guide to Growing Herbs

I have compiled a list of specific herbs in Appendix I, the best methods to propagate them and what kind of environment they grown best in.

And finally, the last appendix provides you with a little more information on preparing wonderful healthy remedies, using specific herbs from your garden. Learn what a tincture is and discover what a poultice is -- and then, more importantly, learn how to make these and use them to help alleviate the minor symptoms of some of the most common health problems.

Enjoying an herb garden is definitely a luxury of life. However, maintaining it shouldn't be at all wearisome. In fact, you'll find once you delve into this book how wonderfully relaxing -- and even therapeutic -- this marvellous hobby can be.

Don't waste another minute! Just get started now deciding on what form your herb garden will take!

Happy Gardening!

Fee

Chapter One:
Why Herbs?

By saying you want to grow herbs
You will inevitably ask "which herbs should I grow?"

Stop! Before you grab that shovel, and before you put a single herb into the ground. Stop and ask yourself exactly why you want an herb garden. You really need to know what the purpose of the herb garden is going to be.

Is the plan to use them both fresh and dried to add to your cooking in order to enhance the flavours? Are you planning on making flavoured oils or vinegars to present to friends and family members as gifts (while keeping a couple stashed for yourself)?

Perhaps you've read or learned that there many natural health benefits of herbs and so you want to grow your own for brewing teas, infusing and making pastes to use to help your minor health conditions?

It certainly matters! Why? Because you need to know which herbs are going to empower your health if that's the aim and not plant herbs designed to embolden your meals.

But beyond just the uses of herbs, you must at some point, decide on the size of your garden. As you journey through this book, you'll see some rather large designs of herb gardens that consume entire back yards. But I'm assuming you won't want to start quite that big (can't say that I blame you!).

If you don't want to "go big" then I'll reveal just how to have smaller container gardens that can be either indoors or out. I'll also show you an option of just growing a small number of herbs, which are manageable, and within reach on your kitchen windowsill.

Whatever you choose, just be prepared to make choices. Of which there will be plenty. These will all sound overwhelming at first. But if you arrive at the start knowing your intentions, even armed with some of your favourite herbs, it certainly won't be such a massive undertaking at all.

And hopefully, as we travel together -- you and I -- you'll discover a few more herbs you hadn't even considered. That really is the true joy of herb gardening -- watching something unexpected spring up.

Culinary herbs.

For many people, using herbs for cooking is the most recognisable and the most useful. Even those who have never used herbs in their life, will have some idea as to what some fresh basil can do to a meal ... the difference some oregano can make in spaghetti sauce ... or how some fresh chives can make a baked potato come to life.

But, then when asked to define a culinary herb, many of us are at quite a loss. Naturally you know what an herb is, however, you probably don't want to give a strict definition. So, here, let me help you out.

Sometimes known as "sweet herbs", culinary herbs are plants that have ripe seeds and tender roots. They smell divine and have an aromatic flavour.

Don't think that you're the first generation to discover some of these herbs -- I hate to disappoint you. As long as mankind (obviously including womankind), has been around it has been literally spicing up cooking with herbs. Some time ago, palaeontologists discovered that the ancient Egyptians used herbs long before the pharaohs began building the pyramids.

The ancient Chinese also turned to the plants in their gardens in order to give their meals flavour and to enhance the appearance.

And of course, you need look no further than the Bible to see how herbs were not only used, but also actually treasured by many. Check out the gospels of Matthew and Luke. In there you'll read that tithes were paid in herbs such as mint, cumin, and other herbs that were deemed valuable.

And in the Old Testament, Isaiah talks about sowing and threshing cumin more that seven hundred years prior to the birth of Christ. And since it's used in the same reference -- and grown in the same fields as -- barley and wheat, you just take for granted that it is used for culinary purposes.

The likes of wheat and barley have remained a staple of cooking but unfortunately, the uses of these specialty herbs have lost the general appeal which is such a shame.

Perhaps there is only one herb that has really kept its status among cooks as a must-have -- and that's parsley. Such herbs as hyssop, rue or horehound are hardly known at all in this day and age, let alone used in the daily cooking.

And this is a shame. Perhaps the meals of today would be a lot more exciting if mankind had kept pace by seriously cultivating some of these herbs, the flavours of them could have been remarkably improved and they would have been used more throughout history.

But mankind's loss can be your gain. Because some herbs are extremely difficult to find, your only option is to grow them yourself. But, today you have the wonderful ability and chance to grow these in your own backyard or on your windowsill.

A Basic Guide to Growing Herbs

Aromatic herbs.

While some of these may include culinary herbs, aromatic herbs are usually grown to be used as additives in products such as perfumes, soaps and other items needing a splendid fragrance.

Not many gardeners cultivate herbs for this reason, so if that's what you are after you will certainly have a stunning effect in your garden.

Aromatic herbs, just like their culinary cousins have a long, rich history that goes just as far back as the culinary plants. The ancient Egyptians, perhaps were the most well known of peoples to use herbs. And they are especially known for the creation of a fragrance called Kyphi. Today, we would classify it as 'incense'. This fragrance was widely used in religious services as part of an overall purification ceremony.

Today you may be growing them to use them intact perhaps to scent your linens or items of clothing. Consider drying these plants -- like marjoram, lovage, rosemary and even basil -- and you'll discover that their precious scents linger for a thankfully long time.

Ornamental herbs.

Then again, your desire to grow herbs may simply be to create a bright environment. No doubt, you've seen the dazzling

A Basic Guide to Growing Herbs

coloured flowers and foliage of many of these wonderful plants. Others have less colour and more pastel or even whitish looking flowers.

These are classified as ornamental herbs. The sole purpose of these herbs is to be decorative. Of course there may be some overlapping. Most culinary herbs are very charming as they grow. Many medicinal herbs are also gorgeous to behold.

Ornamental herbs may be beautiful not so much because of their colours, but for the texture of their leaves. These plants make perfect additions for a balcony or to line your flowerbed.

And if your main purpose is for ornamental -- or decorative -- reasons you may never even harvest these plants.

If you're considering adding herbs to your world for this reason then valerian -- also a very valuable medicinal herb -- is a perfect choice. It has beautiful crimson blossoms. Other good choices are borage and chicory, with their blue (edible) flowers. But don't overlook other herbs that could add delightful colour including chives, variegated thyme and mint lavender.

Another perfect example of an ornamental herb is a type of oregano called the Dittany of Crete. Forming a low mound and producing leaves with fine silvery hairs, this plant was certainly not created to add flavour to any meal -- it was created to be admired!

Medicinal herbs.

Perhaps of all the classifications of herbs, the most interesting, historically, is that of medicinal herbs. Our ancestors at one time treasured these plants. Sometimes they were the only thing that stood between them and death. Long ago, when medical knowledge was either nonexistent or in its infancy, every family had at least one amateur herbalist in its family tree.

Herbal medicine is, without a doubt, the oldest form of 'healthcare' known to the man. No matter how far back in time you travel, you can't find one culture throughout history that didn't use some plant to treat the ill members of its society.

Even primitive humans at the very least observed and appreciated the many different kinds of plants that were available to them to help them heal family and relatives. It's a pity we don't have some record of how the first man (or perhaps more appropriately woman) realised that plants possessed that healing power.

However they discovered it, palaeontologists have found evidence of their use. In one example some thoughtful relative had tucked a few herbs beside the bones of a Stone Age-era man in Iraq. The most notable herbs buried with him were marshmallow root and hyacinth and yarrow.

Today marshmallow root is used to soothe inflammations -- like a sore throat. Hyacinth is used as a diuretic, which encourages tissues to release any excess water they may be retaining. While yarrow is a cold and fever remedy that was just about ubiquitous in its use prior to the synthesis of aspirin.

The ancient Chinese knew their herbs!

The Chinese emperor Shen Nong circa twoseventhreefive BC (when you talk about history that long ago sometimes it's difficult to be extremely precise!) wrote a treatise about the amazing knowledge that was around at the time.

In this treatise, still used to this very day, he recommended an herb called Ma Huang. Its Western name is ephedra. He explains this herb as an excellent remedy to alleviate the signs of respiratory distress. Oh, and did I mention, he did this nearly two and a half thousand years before the birth of Christ.

Today, we have a medication called Ephedrine that is extracted from this herb. It is widely used as a decongestant. It is called pseudoephedrine in its synthetic form and you can find it in many allergy sinus and cold-relief medications today. Hard to believe that nearly five thousand years ago this plant was recognised as a potential healer.

A Basic Guide to Growing Herbs

It's very possible; from the little that the historians have been able to piece together, our ancestors deciphered the plants' healing powers by simply watching the actions of the animals around them.

While for the most part the passing on of this information is strictly oral in nature you'll find several herbalists who recorded some information. This happened mainly in the monasteries because many monks, priests and nuns were very adept at medicinal herbalism.

More likely than not, the specific knowledge of these herbs were passed down from one generation to another. You can hear a grandmother teaching her granddaughter as they work in the herb garden,

"You want to be sure to pick this plant when it's at its greenest. And use this one here when you get a headache. But you'll only require the leaves and stems. Now this herb, dear, you will only need to pick the flowers."

If you're already a budding herbalist then you will know which plants to use for which health problem. No doubt you will also know which part of the plant you'll need such as the leaves, flowers, steams or even the fruits from certain plants and especially their roots to relieve symptoms or to even prevent certain health conditions from ever occurring.

Many a prescription drug derived from herbs.

It is strange to know that many in the medical community look down on the use of herbs. They even regard them as foolish and even dangerous. The irony is that many of today's most effective prescription drugs started off as herbs. What the scientists did was isolate the active ingredients and then recreate them synthetically.

Even the revered -- and most versatile -- aspirin began as the bark of the white willow tree. Scientists then distinguished exactly what made the willow so remarkably valuable. They then synthetically reproduced that particular ingredient and the world's most popular over-the-counter drug was developed: aspirin.

Before the discovery and widespread use of antibiotics, the herb Echinacea – which you may know better as the purple coneflower -- was one of the most widely prescribed medicines in the United States.

Today it's making a comeback for its outstanding ability to help boost the immune system. Many people now take this herb via a capsule or tablet throughout the rough, winter months in order to fend off colds and flu. And, today's modern research has confirmed this plants ability to bolster your immune system. It is the active ingredients in this herb that actually stimulates the production of the much-needed disease-fighting white blood cells.

So what's the bottom line to all of this? Well, if you plan on growing herbs for their medicinal or healing qualities, you'll not only want to know which herbs can help alleviate specific symptoms, but you'll want to learn exactly how to use these herbs.

We've already mentioned the herb Echinacea and this is, in fact one of the easiest of all medicinal herbs to grow. Not only that, but it is also perhaps one of the prettiest. This flower, which is native to the central and eastern United States, resembles a large daisy in its composition. They have a long period of blooming making them a nice resident in your garden.

The Echinacea plant begins to bloom in the spring continues to spread its colour throughout the summer and even carries on into to fall months. It is a hardy plant, not only handling a very hot summer but can also survive droughts.

And they just look so gorgeous anywhere you want to plant them either in the middle of a garden, along its border, in with a rock garden or even in containers.

If you choose Echinacea, just keep in mind it's a tall plant growing to a maximum height of a little more than two to four feet (just over a metre). But the shorter version, Pixie Meadowbrite Coneflower, grows to only a height of a foot and half or so. That's a true dwarf and you'll love its abundance of

A Basic Guide to Growing Herbs

pink flowers. It looks even better still if you mix that strain with another small one, Kim Knee High Coneflower, which has purplish-pink flowers and dense foliage.

Now it's one thing to admire their beauty and fragrance but how do I use medicinal or healing herbs I'm growing? If you're interested in growing herbs you may already have an idea of what are the best ways to prepare them in order to receive the maximum amount of natural healing.

If you're not quite that far in your research or you've just stumbled upon this while reading about other uses of herbs, then read up about some of the really brilliant ways you can use herbs to help improve your health -- sometimes without resorting to harsh chemically based prescription drugs.

Once you're growing your own herbs, then you have full on freedom to use them in a variety of ways. In the back of this book is an appendix in the on how to effectively use your newly grown medicinal herbs. There you will find step-by-step procedures for preparing your plants in a variety of ways.

Tea Time!

If you enjoy a nice, quality cup of tea, then I'm picking that you wouldn't mind growing your own plants to steep and enjoy in the mid-afternoon, or maybe even a relaxing cup before bedtime.

A Basic Guide to Growing Herbs

If you decide to plant herbs to enjoy a "tea garden" you can rest assured that you will be following in the footsteps of many who have gone before you. The tradition dates back literally thousands of years. Both the Chinese and Japanese cultures have been doing this for as long as anyone can remember.

There's just something about the composition of the Orient that tea is a part and parcel of the meditative process. Not only did they drink tea, but also these cultures created niches to enjoy this beverage undisturbed.

But that doesn't mean the Europeans didn't have their share of tea gardens. The most well known of the tea drinkers, the English, created formal and cottage gardens exclusively for the growing of various teas.

If you love tea, then without a doubt, you have probably wanted to experience what it would be like if, for once your tea leaves didn't come packaged in a box, surrounded by a bag.

Now that you have a better idea of the different types of herbs you can work out why you'd like to start an herb garden then continue your thoughts with what herbs you'd like to grow. This seems like the only logical transition. So let's get on with the next chapter, which is all about which herbs to plant.

A Basic Guide to Growing Herbs

Chapter Two:
Which Herbs?

Now that you've established the purpose of your herb garden, you can make some choices about exactly which herbs you'll include.

Yes, you're definitely excited now. You can't wait to start your garden. You can smell the aromatic plants growing in your back yard or even closer, your kitchen windowsill. You can even visualise yourself reaching for some fresh herbs to add to your ingredients as you prepare your dinner.

But, as you drive to the nursery to choose your plants, you're still puzzled about exactly which ones to grow. I can understand your confusion. When I first began planting herbs, I experienced the same uncertainty.

That's why I've developed what I call my "Top Ten List of Must-Grow Herbs." There are two lists – one for culinary and one for medicinal. These are not only some of the most commonly used herbs in cooking/medicinal but they represent some of the easiest ones to grow. I've also provided with this list, what type of soil and other essential growing conditions you need for success.

A Basic Guide to Growing Herbs

Top 10 culinary herbs.

With this list in hand on your first trip to the nursery, you're bound to have success in finding what not only works in your yard but choices that will mesh well with your taste buds.

1. Basil

Basil is the best herb for pesto, hands down. Its leaves have a warm and spicy flavour. You need to only add a small amount of this delightful herb in such dishes as soups, salads and sauces. Basil is also particular suited, by the way, to season any dish with tomato flavouring. Great topped on pizza or pasta.

You'll want to start your basil plants early in the spring, preferably in a greenhouse or a sun-drenched windowsill. Early in the summer transplant this herb to your garden. Or, if you have the courage, sow basil seeds directly into the garden early in the spring. Or you may want to try your hand at both methods, just in case those seeds don't catch.

2. Chives

Who doesn't love some fresh chives on a hot, newly baked potato? If you're as mad about this herb as I am, then you've already noticed that chives have a mildly onion taste. This makes them an excellent addition to salads, sandwich spreads and sauces. And, oh, by the way, don't restrict chives to just the baked potato. Taste how in adds a little zing to your salads as

A Basic Guide to Growing Herbs

well. As a bonus you can use the chive flowers which looks great in a salad!

If you plan on growing chives from starter plants, then you'll want to get these into your garden in the early spring. And you'll want to give these plants plenty of room. My recommendation is to plant them a good nine to twelve inches (thirty cm) from each other.

If you plan to plant the chives seeds, then plant them in the fall or the spring, digging down a good half inch (one cm) and setting the seeds in rows that are spaced about twelve inches (thirty cm) apart.

Another variety of chives is the garlic flavoured one so you might like to plant both.

3. Coriander

Now here's a versatile herb. Its versatility is so great that different parts of this plant are known as different herbs. Grinding the dried seeds means you're using coriander. Using the leaves to add to some Indian or Asian dishes? You're actually using cilantro.

And of course you can use the roots of coriander as well. If you can't use them right away, don't worry you can freeze these.

A Basic Guide to Growing Herbs

They can be used to flavour soups. Or chop the roots and serve with avocados. You'll find this deliciously delightful!

Even a novice herbalist should have no problem growing coriander from seeds (I know I did it my first time around and there was no novice who was more naïve and at a loss than I!)

Sow these seeds in the early spring. Dig a hole about quarter inch (half cm) in depth. Plant them in rows that are just about a foot (thirty cm) apart. Once the seedlings appear, you'll want to thin them down some, making sure they're at least six inches (fifteen cm) from the other.

4. Dill

Here's another herb that you can use both the seeds and the leaves. Both of these parts have a sharp, slightly bitter taste. (But then who among us doesn't know the taste of dill?)

Whether you use it fresh or dried, you'll find it a most tasty addition to a lot of different dishes. Don't be afraid to add it to salads and soups as well. And many people use the leaves in potatoes. Another way to enjoy the unique taste of this herb is to sprinkle a little dill on sliced cucumbers for use as a sandwich filling.

Dill is another easy plant to grow from seed. Plant your seeds in the early spring, about quarter inch (half cm) deep. You'll

# A Basic Guide to Growing Herbs

want to make sure you leave at least nine inches (twenty-two cm) between these seeds. Once the seedlings appear, be sure to thin them, keeping them those nine inches (twenty-two cm) apart.

5. Fennel

Many individuals love to use fennel in soups and salads as well as pastas and lentils.

The leaves themselves have a sweet flavour. The seeds, though, have a sharper flavour to them.

Want to try your hand at growing fennel from seeds? These are easy enough to do so. Plant your seeds in groups of three or four about mid-spring. You'll dig a small hole about a quarter inch (half cm) deep. Place the seeds about one and half feet (forty-five cm) apart. Once these grow into seedlings, you'll want to thin them.

6. Mint

Ah, what would an herb garden be without mint? Mint is an essential herb whether you plant a culinary herb or medicinal herb garden (or a little of both!).

Use the leaves to brew into a nice, satisfying hot tea. Or use them to add a dash of sunshine to cold drinks as well. Mint is

A Basic Guide to Growing Herbs

also a great garnish. Spearmint, specifically, is used to make a mint sauce or jelly.

You'll want to start planting your mint in the autumn or spring. You'll also have the best results if you begin with the actual roots of the plants. Plant four inches (ten cm) to six inches (fifteen cm) pieces of the root. Make sure they're about two inches (five cm) deep and a good twelve inches (thirty cm) apart.

Then make sue you water these guys well. Check the roots occasionally. They are quite aggressive. By this, I mean they seem to easily overtake the roots of neighbouring plants. You can easily prevent this by sinking boards or brinks about one-foot deep around the beds.

You may also take an extra precaution when you first plant them. Plant them in the garden bed itself, but enclose a plastic bucket with no bottom around it. That keeps them contained for a specific depth.

7. Parsley

For me, parsley brings back memories of my grandmother. She had parsley planted everywhere. And she used in everything, but especially in soup. As a youngster we lived next door to my grandmother. When my mother had planned to make soup, she would send me over to my grandmother to retrieve a supply of parsley.

In addition to soups, parsley makes a great addition to just about any meal you can think of an especially great in salads so it is eaten raw.

If you're planning on growing the plant from seed, start planting them in mid-spring if you want to use the herb in the summer. Plant the seeds in mid-summer if you want fresh autumn and winter parsley.

Before you plant the seeds, you'll need to soak them overnight. When this plant reaches seedling stage thin the bed out and make sure the plants are around ten inches (twenty-five cm) apart.

8. Sage

Most think of sage as being the herb that is added to onion to make stuffing. However, sage goes with many other dishes such as polenta, beans, lentils, apples and pineapple. In fact you can actually even get a pineapple sage plant, which is wonderfully aromatic. You can infuse honey with sage as well as olive oil and to beat everything you can deep-fry the leaves to serve as an appetizer.

A Basic Guide to Growing Herbs

Sage is another plant that can easily be grown from its seeds. You'll want to start planting in the early spring if you plan on doing this. If you prefer, though, you can be starter plants from your local nursery. If you're going this route, you can wait until mid-spring to set these out. Just be sure to plant them about a foot (thirty cm) apart.

9. Tarragon

If you think anything like I do, you hear the word tarragon and immediately think vinegar. And it is a great flavouring for vinegar. Up until now you may have run to the store to buy your tarragon vinegar. But consider waking up one morning, picking some tarragon from your garden, placing it in vinegar, steeping it for two to three weeks and then enjoying your own homemade tarragon vinegar!

But vinegar is just the start of how this plant can dramatically change your eating habits, given a little time and experimentation. The leaves of this herb have a taste that is something akin to anise, which makes it ideal for a variety of dishes. Try placing the leaves in soups and stews. From there you can experiment with salads.

But don't let your use of this versatile herb stop there. Think vegetable dishes as well as sauces. Let your imagination soar when it comes to your use of tarragon.

A Basic Guide to Growing Herbs

When you grow this herb though, steer clear of trying to grow it from seeds. You just won't have any luck. Instead, visit your local nursery and buy some small plants. You'll dig and plant these in early spring, making sure they have lots of room to grow. In this case, give them at least eighteen inches (forty-five cm) from another. Yeah, these guys get pretty big.

10. Thyme

Yes, thyme. And no, I have no idea why we have to spell it this way. But despite its awkward spelling, and its fame as a starring role in an old Simon and Garfunkel song, thyme is a must grow for any self-respecting herbalist.

Thyme is a great seasoning for just about any dish. You can sprinkle chopped fresh leaves (you can use dried as well) over roasted vegetables before you even put them in the oven.

This herb also goes to work for you in various other capacities too. It is great on potatoes, tomatoes, lima beans, rice and summer squash. Nice in soups too. You'll be pleasantly surprised when you start experimenting with thyme.

I even know one person who brews her thyme to make tea. She just adds a bit of rosemary and a sprig of mint to go with it!

Go ahead, you can start this herb from seeds. Sometime in mid-spring make shallow rows for the seeds about a foot (thirty cm) apart. When the thyme seedlings are established, you'll then thin them out placing them about six inches (fifteen cm) from each other.

If you don't feel up to starting thyme from seeds, you'll want to plant your nursery-bought seedlings about mid-spring -- again keeping them at least six inches (fifteen cm) apart, preferably nine inches (twenty-two cm) if you have the room.

Growing medicinal herbs? Top ten healing herbs.

So you want to try to hand at a few of those herbs you've read about -- and used in various forms -- to help improve your health. But, you haven't fully decided about all the plants to be included in your garden.

While you're making that decision, let me supply you with some of the most popular of the herbs. Not only have I included the herb, and the growing conditions it likes the best, I've also included how it may improve your health.

Here's my "top ten list" of medicinal herbs for gardeners. Some of these are fairly common, some of them you may not have heard about unless you know your healing herbs -- and a few may come as a surprise to you!

A Basic Guide to Growing Herbs

1. Nettles

Easy to grow, the nettles plant family has been used for generations (and then some) as an effective aid against inflammation due to allergies, arthritis and even lupus. It's also been used successful as a tonic for helping alleviate the symptoms of anaemia.

And no wonder it's effective. It's rich in iron and vitamin C. Herbalists not only use the leaves of this plant, but they also put the roots to good use treating symptoms as well.

But that's not all because the plant is abundant in various antioxidants, as well as flavonoids -- all health-giving properties that medicine is only now beginning to appreciate.

When harvesting this plant for medicinal purposes, you'll want to be sure that the ones you choose are "sticky." This indicates the presence of resin, which is its active healing ingredient.

Sometimes called stinging nettles, you'll want to be sure to wear gloves when you harvest this plant. It packs a good sting, while harmless, still hurts. And you'll find that you can harvest nettles several times throughout the year.

Nettle is also a plant that "reseeds" itself, which is wonderful because you'll have access to it all year round. Be careful where you plant this herb though. If not pruned back this plant grows to over six feet (182 cm), which means it may just squeeze out some others in your garden.

If you begin your first season by growing nettles from seeds, be sure to germinate them for ten to fourteen days even before you place them in the ground. Keep the seeds at room temperature. Start your planting in the spring.

Then transplant the seedlings to an area where they receive full sun and just partial shade. Keep the plants at least eight inches (twenty cm) to twelve inches (thirty cm) from each other.

2. Calendula

This plant, with its bright flowers, is an important part of any healer's garden. Never heard of it? Ah, but I'm betting you've seen it. You probably called it a marigold. That's right! It's also called the calendula and is one of the most versatile healing herbs available.

Starting with its striking orange bloom, which is used by many as a soothing skin wash, a tea and a salve, this plant is a staple in my herb garden.

The flower is also edible, so feel free to brighten up your next salad by garnishing it with the calendula. The overall gentle healing qualities of this plant makes it a great ingredient for --

you guessed it -- diaper salves as well as other baby-related skincare items.

Scientific studies show that the calendula may actually help stimulate your immune system and support improved microcirculation -- that is the circulation of your blood right down to those tiny capillaries!

The calendula is easy to grow from seeds. Plant the seeds early in the spring and cover them lightly with about a quarter inch (half cm) of garden soil. Once the seedlings pop up, you'll want to transplant them so they are about fifteen inches (thirty-eight cm) from the other.

You'll discover that they germinate early as well as grow quite quickly. And you'll be pleasantly surprised they produce their very first blooms by mid-summer.

The best part of this wonderful plant is that it reseeds itself. Once you've planted them the first time, they will grow for years as long as you don't disturb them.

Calendula love rich, well-drained soil, but they're hardy and they can live in just about any type of soil. While these may sound like the perfect herb -- a gorgeous flower, many healing qualities and a hardiness to survive just about any terrain -- the plant does have one drawback. They attract insects.

Aphids seem especially fond of this plant. But don't let that discourage you. There are different organic sprays and washes you can use. Before you bring them indoors, make sure you inspect thoroughly for the presence of these insects.

3. Burdock

You may be hard pressed to find this herb in most gardens, but including it in yours will make your garden all that much more distinctive. Sometimes this herb is referred to as gobo, but if you haven't heard it as either name, I'm not really surprised.

Burdock tea moreover, is beneficial for your gastrointestinal tract as well as used by many to boost a slacking appetite. Herbalists have also used this tea to help restore liver function.

Though not native to this country, burdock grows freely in many areas. It was brought over by the original settlers during early colonial at times.

Most people start burdock from seed. Start planting in the early spring -- the earlier the better in fact. Cover the seeds with quarter inch (half cm) to half inch (one cm) of fine garden soil or seed starting soil. If the water seems dry when you plant, then you'll want to water it as well.

The seeds germinate quickly, so you should notice some sprouts in about four to seven days. Take the seedlings and thin them until they're about three inches (seven and half cm) apart, in rows separated by at least two feet (sixty cm). This plant prefers the full sun, but is hardy enough to tolerate some shade as well.

If you're considering growing burdock then you also need to consider the soil in which you place it. This plant needs a rich well-drained soil. The soil itself should be loose and definitely free from rocks and stones.

And that's not just on the surface. Be sure that the area below this plant, for at least several feet in depth is rock-free. This allows the burdock's root to take hold securely. And it does have a big, strong root.

And yes, you can eat this herb too. Pick the leaves when they are quite tender, then cook them just like you would spinach.

If you're planning on using the roots as a medicinal tool, then you'll have to wait for a while. They take a good long time to grow. Some herbalists say you need to wait about one hundred days. Don't pick the roots before they're two feet (sixty cm) long. Then you simply peel them. You may either eat the root raw or cook it. Many people use the root in soups, salads and even in stir-fry dinners.

4. Chamomile

This is perhaps one of the best known of all the healing herbs, thanks to the commercialisation, marketing and popularity of chamomile tea. You may already buy and drink this tea prior to going to sleep at night, or when your nerves seem agitated. The plant is best known for its calming effects on the human body.

And more recently, scientific studies coming from England are conferring additional healing powers on this already beloved plant. Drinking chamomile tea may do more than just make you sleepy. It could also boost your immune system, making you more resistant to colds and the flu as well as other infections.

But did you realise that you can grow this fascinating herb and make your own tea? And use the plant in several other ways to help your system?

This herb is easy to grow from seed. It loves the full sun and does well in average soil -- but really thrives in a rich environment. You'll want to plant your seeds in the spring. Once they grow into seedlings, thin them to fifteen to eighteen inches (thirty eight to forty-five cm) of each other.

They require little care. When harvesting this herb, you'll want to wait until the flowers reach their peak bloom. For remedies, you can use the plant either fresh or dried. Drying of the flowers is quite easy by the way. Simply spread them out in a cool and well-ventilated place. That's all you need to do!

Use the flowers to brew the tea. You can also add the flowers to other kinds of tea to make a light and refreshing blend. You can serve this hot or cold, or be imaginative and serve this mixture in a punch.

5. Echinacea

Definitely give this healing herb a chance in your healing garden. You've no doubt heard about the wonderful properties of this plant. Echinacea has been noted for the last several years as a powerful booster for your immune system. Many individuals take this herb in capsule or tablet form as a supplement to avoid contracting colds and the flu, especially during the winter months.

This plant, with its large, bright flower is also known as the purple coneflower. There are three distinct varieties of Echinacea: Echinacea pallid, Echinacea angustifolia and Echinacea pupuea. All three have similar medicinal effects.

Many herbalists also use this plant for respiratory infections. In Europe, it's not unusual for medicinal doctors to prescribe this to their patients for a variety of remedies.

You might think with all these wonderfully effective health benefits, Echinacea would be near impossible to grow (aren't we conditioned to believe there's a catch behind every good thing?). Well nothing could be further from the truth. It's actually quite easy to grow. One of the most amazing aspects of their success is their tolerance for dry conditions.

And you can actually grow this amazing plant from seed with little trouble. Plant the seeds when your soil reaches between fifty five - seventy degrees Fahrenheit (twelve – twenty two degrees C) in the spring.

You need do nothing more initially than sow the seeds on the surface. Within ten to twenty days, you should notice the seeds germinating. Once this happens, then you'll cover them with about one-eighth of an inch of soil.

When they reach the seedling stage, you'll want to thin the plants so they're about eighteen to twenty-four inches (forty-five - sixty cm) apart.

This plant prefers shade to full sun. You may also want to test your soil's pH balance before planting your seeds. This plant prefers neutral soil, with a rating of six to eight.

Echinacea bloom from June to October. And, oh yes, they attract the most beautiful of butterflies! Even if you don't use the plant for health reasons, its presence in your garden lifts your spirit when you watch the butterflies hover around it!

6. Lavender

No herbal healing garden would be complete without at least a small place dedicated to the lavender. Lavender is to healing pain what Echinacea is to the immune system: indispensible!
One of the most effective topical creams I've ever used had lavender as its main herbal ingredient!

The health benefits of lavender are many. In addition to relieving pain, it's noted for it relaxing effects -- the remarkable ability to relieve anxiety. Partly because of this ability, it is used as a "cure" for insomnia as well as a muscle relaxant.

But beyond that, there may be some hard scientific evidence that lavender may also help support healthy blood pressure levels.

If you're not familiar with what the plant looks like, you'll recognise it once you see it. It has needle-like, foliage that's bluish-grey in colour, topped with violet-blue slender-looking flowers. The long-blooming flowers are sure to delight you throughout the entire growing season.

A Basic Guide to Growing Herbs

This plant is, thankfully, drought tolerant, making it easy to care for. Don't try to start this herb from seed though. Your best bet is to go to your nursery to buy small plants that were cuttings from another plant.

If you insist on trying your hand at starting lavender from seed, then grow the seeds in small pots early in the spring. The drawback with this method is that the seeds may die before they fully germinate.

Even if you get some seeds to survive, the next obstacle you need to overcome is the slow sprouting of the seeds -- in some cases more than two weeks. This invites the growth of fungus on the small plants. In some cases, these poor things actually rot before they get the chance to grow.

Once you have a successful plant in your garden, make sure it's in an area that is well drained.

7. Lemon Balm

A healing herb garden shouldn't be without Lemon Balm. Originally native to southern Europe, it is now found everywhere on the globe.

Its medicinal traits are similar to those of the mint. It produces a positive effect on the digestive system and is also used to relieve pain and discomfort that usually comes with indigestion. Individuals who suffer from anxiety, nervousness as well as mild insomnia also use this plant with much success.

The most common method of using the medicinal healing powers of this plant is through steeping the leaves for tea.

Part of the mint family, lemon balm grows to be about a foot to a foot and a half tall, and has a small two-lipped flower that blooms in the late summer. And as you might guess from its name, its leaves have a definite aroma and flavour of lemon.

This marvellous plant is really quite easy to grow outside. It actually grows in clumps and then spreads itself via its seeds. You'll find that in the winter, the stems of the plant will die off, but don't worry about that. They shoot up again on their own the following spring.

You can also start growing lemon balm simply by taking stem cuttings or, if you prefer, you can grow them from seed. But I'm warning you, if the seeds find the right environment, you'll soon have lemon balm everywhere! Of course, there are worse things to have in your garden.

When you're planting the herb initially, the plants should be placed about twelve or fifteen inches (thirty – thirty-eight cm) apart to give them plenty of "elbowroom."

8. St. John's Wort

St. John's Wort is not a native to the United States, but today you can find it growing along the roadside in many regions where the climate is mild. This prolific plant normally blooms from late May through to September, depending on the climate.

In fact, its name comes to us because of the timing of its flowering. It once was believed that the plant bloom on the birthday of St. John the Baptist, June twenty-four.

You probably are already familiar with this plant as a healing herb. Lately it not only has been recommended by just about everyone, but scrutinized closely by the medical community. It is best known in the treatment of depression.

By all means, this is one of those perfect plants to try starting by seed. But if you're not up to that challenge, you can also propagate it through small cuttings or by rooting. No matter how you choose to start the plant, you'll eventually want to give it at least quite a bit of space so they don't crowd each other out. You can thin them when the seedlings are about two inches tall.

For optimum growing it really doesn't matter where you plant this herb. It'll grow just about anywhere. It grows well in full to partial sun, but also tolerates the shade well. It grows best though in moist light soils.

A Basic Guide to Growing Herbs

9. Feverfew

Perhaps the name is not familiar to you but I'm sure the flower is. Feverfew, known for centuries as a natural cure for a migraine headache, has a flower that closely resembles the daisy. White petals with yellow centres, accent the green serrated leaves of this plant. If left to its own devices, these gorgeous flowers can grow to a height of nearly two feet.

In addition to migraines, many individuals say that using this plant has helped their arthritis and rheumatism.

And the most beautiful aspect of this amazing plant -- it'll bloom just about all summer long.

Feverfew grows in just about any type of soil, as it really isn't a fussy plant at all. This makes it perfect to place between stones or pavers on your walkways and paths.

Go ahead; definitely try starting this plant from seeds. You'll probably have good luck with this method. If you're not quite brave enough, that's all right too. Feverfew will catch on and grow from cuttings just as well.

10. Valerian

Never considered this plant as part of your herbal garden? Perhaps you should give it a second look. Oh, yes, I know that the first year or two of growing these plants you're not even going to find one flower on them.

And yes, I know they won't be the most pleasantly fragrant herb in your garden. But if you're a serious herbalist, you'll probably want to include this herb anyway.

Why? It appears to be on the versatile healing herb list. But you really don't have to take my word for it. Herbalists and other healers throughout the ages have been using this plant for a variety of illnesses and health conditions.

Valerian is said to be a great natural treatment for anxiety, as well as nervous tension and restlessness. It has also been said to help relieve stomach cramps and various digestive disorders. And that's just the start of what herbalists like about this plant.

Don't let its lack of flowers for the first several years deter you from growing this. Its foliage alone -- without any blooms -- will add texture and colour to your garden.

The best method of starting your own plants is by separating the roots and then planting these separately. Another advantage to growing valerian is that it really isn't particular about where it grows. It can grow almost anywhere.

A Basic Guide to Growing Herbs

If you've got a damp area in your garden where nothing else grows, try placing a couple plants here. Or if you have some rocky spots that look empty, valerian plants will fill those nicely too!

Chapter Three:
Design A Garden

Got your herbs all lined up in a row, ready to plant? Now it's time to design your garden. Whether it takes up your entire yard or just a small square, the more thought you put into it, the more beautiful it will be.

Did you ever think of yourself as an "architect"? No? Well, go look into the mirror and introduce yourself to the new you. Now you are about to be the architect and the creative vision behind your very own herb garden.

Don't worry! We'll take it slow. But, you're still taking an active hand in the designing of exactly where your garden goes. You'll be utterly amazed at just how easy it is.

Most people (and you might not be one of them, I understand) start their hobby on a modest scale. They begin by dedicating for the herbs, an area of around twenty by four feet (twenty by one-half metres). And then they break this area up into twelve by eighteen inch (thirty by forty-five cm) plots -- each different herb assigned its own special plot.

Just a quick hint that is something to think about before you go shopping for these plants. Within this space, it's not unusual to see parsley and purple basil as border plants. These are not only placed in a spot that's handy to pick, but they're colourful and add beauty to this spot in your yard.

But even I'm getting ahead of myself now. Because if you really want a well-designed garden, then you need to pick up a pencil and several pieces of graph paper. Yes, you're about to outline -- and literally design -- your very own herb garden.

And no, it's really not nearly as frightening as it sounds. In fact, it's quite fun. After all, if Ralph Waldo Emerson is correct (and who am I to argue with a dead writer) then every thing we see in this world started as a thought -- and your herb garden is no different.

The best way to transfer a thought into a reality -- write it down. And so we will. Let's face it, you know that your herb garden is already blooming and growing wildly in your imagination even as I write this.

Long before any digging is done, you're planting the seeds of your garden as you visualise where your basil will live, whether you'll put your valerian in the left corner or in the middle of the garden ... well you get the idea.

And don't worry. You definitely don't have to be an artist to sketch a garden -- especially if you cheat just a little as I suggested earlier: use graph paper. This will keep things in perspective for you.

A Basic Guide to Growing Herbs

Before you rush in to even sketching though, there are five **MUST-ASK** questions only you can answer. And yes, these questions have a direct bearing on the eventual look, feel and overall effect of your garden:

1. How large of a space do you have for your garden (don't be ashamed to say just a small balcony in the middle of a large city!)

2. How much sun does it get? Is it predominantly sunny or are there more total hours of shade?

3. Which growing zone are you in? (You can find this out by going to: Google and typing into the search -- Find my growing zone *your country*

4. How are you planning to spend time in your garden? How do you intend to use your garden?

5. What type of soil do you have?

Now that your ideal herb garden is beginning to gel in your mind, you can transfer those tentative ideas onto paper. And do remember you're putting this on paper and with pencil -- not chiselling it into stone.

What does that means? It means that you are going to have an eraser right along side your paper, because you're bound to change your mind at least once, if not multiple times, during this process.

To keep you accurate, each square on your graph paper equals one foot (thirty cm) in your eventual garden. This makes it super-simple to transfer the ideas into the physical world later.

In addition to this, you may also want to have some type of circular template so you can easily trace around it. Some plants, shrubs and even trees are usually drawn as various circles in a sketched garden design.

For example, let's say tucked among your herb garden you have a three-foot (ninety cm) wide dwarf shrub. You'll need a circle encompassing three squares on your graph paper.

Now, if you really want to nail down your imagination, have some coloured pencils lined up to use as well. How else are you going to know what *colour* herbs to place next to each other?

Planting your garden on paper.

Seeding your imagination

Step one:

This exercise is valuable because it allows you to actually lay out and "try on" any number of garden plans. Are you at a loss

A Basic Guide to Growing Herbs

of just where to start? Begin by showing what you already have, those things that in all practicality just aren't going to move -- like fully-grown trees!

Other immovable structures you may have to work around include fences and backyard decks or patios.

Step two:

Next, decide which views you'd like to create. This means what the overall look of your garden will be. Included in this process will be determining aspects about the area you'd like to "soften" up a bit or perhaps hide altogether.

Are you looking forward to sitting at your kitchen table, sipping that first cup of coffee in the morning and seeing ....? Perhaps Echinacea blooming? Or maybe Hawthorne growing? Even the purplish round chubby head of a chives bloom staring back at you?

Or would you prefer sitting there drinking your coffee, while at the same time, you drink in the simply luscious scents of some aromatic herbs?

Now that you've taken that step, continue with what you'll see from your window or patio in all four seasons. Obviously in spring and summer, you'll be looking at foliage and blooms. But what do you want to see in autumn? Do you really want to look at ... well, nothing but worn out flowers?

A Basic Guide to Growing Herbs

Step three:

Draw the lines that are to be borders of your planting areas. Remember that each square represents one foot (thirty cm). Keep a ruler next to you as a visual reminder if you have to (I do, because I'm just a member of the "measurement challenged" community). Leave room for the layering of different types of herbs, like your perennials and your shrubs.

Step four:

Your next step is to draw in those large immoveable objects in your garden that you know, right from the start; you'll need to work around. You know, that tree over there, the fence in the back -- those types of things.

Step five:

Now it's time to give serious consideration to the types of herbs you'd like to have where. And be precise about this. Start with perennial herbs; try to keep these in groups of around three to five plants in an area. You'll appreciate this piece of advice once they've bloomed.

This is the fun part of the design approach, the part where your seeds of imagination really can germinate into a beautiful and fragrant herb garden. And I'm certainly not about to stop you now!

A Basic Guide to Growing Herbs

Idea-less in your garden?

Don't tell me you're sitting there without a clue of what to choose. You've got all those magazines in front of you, all of those herb catalogues. Even the list I've given you earlier on in this book. Well, let me give you a helpful hint or two.

Leaf through those magazines again. Yes, you don't have a back yard like they're showing. But what is it about those gardens that are especially appealing, what keeps drawing you back to this garden or that garden. Jot it down. Now look at a few other magazines. Go to your local library; visit a larger bookstore in search of magazines even go to thrift stores where magazines are usually free. It doesn't matter how out-of-date they are, herb gardens don't date.

Perhaps you're just considering container gardening? Then why not pay attention to your local coffee shop? You know the one. It has those container plants grouped so nicely. Get some inspiration from them.

Go online and check out some websites. Here you'll get a wide variety of ideas of what to place in your garden, depending on your purpose for planting.

Types of herb gardens.

Until I gained an interest in herbs, I really had no idea that there were different categories of herb garden designs. But did I learn and quickly. And indeed you can find entire books devoted to the exact design and layout of gardens, which plants are placed where -- and sometimes even a detailed reasoning why.

I would be remiss if I didn't mention them to you. But don't feel that just because you're starting a new hobby that you have to redesign your entire backyard. Not unless you really wanted a good excuse to.

Much of the design of your garden, in fact, depends on the amount of shade your yard receives -- and where -- the amount of sun available for the herbs, the type of soil you have and just what type of herbs you'd like to grow.

But, still it's interesting and fun to learn more about the design of various gardens and their origins.

Formal.

No, this doesn't mean you and your guests must dress in tuxedoes in order to enter the garden. The layouts of garden actually date back to medieval and Renaissance Europe. And if you visit public botanical gardens today you'll discover that we are still influenced by these practices.

Of course, we don't know what average Joe "Serf" and his family planted or how they planted them. No doubt they were arranged in an order that emphasized usefulness and ease of access.

But we do know that monasteries and the royal palaces and the gardens of the upper classes were more defined -- and followed certain ideas.

In fact, one of the oldest renditions of a formal herb garden that is known dates back to the ninth century. As far as historians know the garden, which was designed for a Benedictine monastery, was never actually constructed (is that exactly the right word for building a garden?).

But the logic behind the plans is amazing. First, the plans include a large, rectangular kitchen garden. And when I say large, I mean large. Some eighteen beds of vegetables and potherbs were anticipated.

Another sixteen beds were to be devoted strictly to the medicinal herbs. And its anticipated location is quite interesting -- right next to the doctor's house near the infirmary.

A Basic Guide to Growing Herbs

Both of these garden plots were to be walled; each one was to be laid out in two parallel rows of rectangular raised beds and each bed was devoted to a single species of herbs. Yes, indeed, the monks knew exactly what they wanted.

This was a basic utilitarian design and is quite typical of monastic life as well as just about any large medieval garden.

Fast-forward some six hundred years later. We have drawings of fifteenth century gardens of rural manors and townhouses. What we know about these is that they were composed of any number of small square or rectangular beds arranged in a simple grid pattern. Paths, with ample room for strolling, connected the various squares.

We still use this general outline to this day. And it is not a bad basic design for an herb garden -- you may even want to consider it. After all, its design is based on ease of use. This design -- species by species -- makes it easy to harvest the medicinal herbs as well as rotate the short-lived crops of salad herbs.

Indeed, this particular design of a formal garden works not only on a visually pleasing level, but also on the utilitarian level.

A Basic Guide to Growing Herbs

Not all medieval gardens were created equal.

But don't think that every garden in that era was laid out exactly like that. Many weren't. Many residents of these vast estates tossed utility out the door and followed their own imaginations.

One gentleman created a garden that featured the lawn in the centre of the yard, and surrounding this in a circular fashion he planted sweet-smelling herbs like basil, rue, and sage. These gardens promoted elements that many of us still promote today when we grow our herbal gardens, elements like intimacy, enclosure and fragrance.

The botanical garden.

This type of garden also originated in the medieval era. And you might be surprised to learn the original intent was a teaching tool. Created by universities to teach their students medicine, these gardens included narrow, rectangular beds much in the medieval fashion. The London Society of Apothecaries in the seventeenth century founded the Chelsea Physic Garden, where the garden beds are still being used today in the original medieval design.

A Basic Guide to Growing Herbs

Medieval gives rise to renaissance.

Ah, the Renaissance, known for a resurgence of ... well, it looks like just about everything. Art wasn't the only item to gain popularity suddenly. The herb garden changed form during this time as well.

It went well beyond the "basic forms' of the medieval version and grew into more complex endeavours. It's as if those who witnessed the unfolding of the art world weren't satisfied to contain the changes to just one area.

Gone suddenly were the neat, rectangular designs that emphasized utility. Now, gardeners designed for beauty. The patterns of herbs grew more complex.

A design called "the knot", still used today in herb gardens, was developed. Decorative interlacing bands of neatly clipped herbs were featured. A geometric design within a square, a rectangle or even a circle was created on the ground.

Each figure in the pattern was then assigned and filled with a single herb, meticulously manicured to maintain the ultimate design.

If spaces were found between these clipped outlines they were filled with gravel or different coloured sand. In the Elizabethan era these gaps were filed with lavender, germander or even santolina (which is a genus of plants in the chamomile tribe within the sunflower family, primarily from the western Mediterranean region.)

The knot garden to this day is still one of the most popular designs. Open just about any book devoted exclusively to garden design and its one of the first designs you'll see.

Devising your culinary herb garden.

"But I don't want to create a huge garden just for herbs," you explain patiently. And that's quite understandable. Thankfully there's really no need to. Why dedicate your time and effort to a process of designing and planting that you really won't enjoy. You see herb growing is all about enjoyment.

So, let me clue you in on a little secret. Herbs -- and culinary herbs especially -- can make themselves at home just about any place in your existing flower garden. Heck, even if you don't have a flower garden now, you can find some place in your yard for an herb here and an herb there. That's just part of the beauty and ease of growing herbs.

Got roses blooming already? Go ahead and place an herb as its neighbour. You may want to place your basil next to those petunias. It's your garden, why not? Already got a small vegetable garden going, by all means intersperse your vegetables with herbs.

A Basic Guide to Growing Herbs

And don't even panic if you've never planted anything before. I know one gentleman who planted catnip along the cement block foundation of his back porch. He wasn't into planting a lot, just four or five plants. The green added wonderful colour and ... okay, so those herbs weren't really for him. His cat appreciated and enjoyed them though -- when he was inside and played with toys filled with catnip. And when the cat was outside it snuggled up next to them.

You get the point. Design is great -- if you enjoy it. But if you're just testing the waters, you may not want to devote that much time to it.

But what if you want to go for a larger look but keep it informal?

Start with the herbs that you know are going to grow taller than the others. These specific ones are sure to "add interest" to the landscape you're laying out. Most of these you'll want to place behind the shorter ones.

In a very real sense, your garden, when completed, looks layered. The shortest plants will be in front, some of them being used as border accents. Choose the plants proportionally to place behind the others. You'll want to see -- and certainly you'll want your visitors to see - all of them. What use would it do to have the parsley hidden behind a larger coriander plant?

You'll be surprised at just how many of the herbs will grow quite large if you allow them and encourage them. Bay laurel, by nature is a large herb. You can encourage this plant to grow a larger trunk, simply by pruning it.

Or you may just let it grow into its natural shape -- many larger main stems -- simply by doing nothing.

Rosemary, normally not a very large plant, can be encouraged to grow bigger. All you need to do is remove its lower branches. You can also allow your garden sage to rise above the rest.

The look still isn't quite what you had in mind? Why not plant certain herbs in their own containers, and then place these in your herb garden. Containers create a pleasing texture to the eye. Not only that, but depending on the type of container and its colour, add a delightful dash of colour to your garden.

The only piece of advice I'd like to give you before you begin is this: place this culinary garden as close to the kitchen as possible. This way your favourite herbs are nearby, not only ready to use but easy to get to. Instead of reaching for the store-bought bottles of dried herbs, you simply step outside your back door and pick a few fresh ones. Does life really get any better than this?

Another piece of advice for gardening with herbs: don't be stingy. Yes, you heard me. Be generous when you plant. Don't plant just one basil plant or one thyme. Plant the different types in groups of three or even five.

Other ideas to keep in mind when you're planting your informal culinary garden include the presence of a path through part of it. This path not only serves as a wonderful mindful meditation road for those of who you are thoughtful. But it serves the larger purpose of providing easy access to all the herbs you choose to pick without trampling through the smaller ones.

Accents in your garden.

No your culinary garden doesn't need to be large, but consider placing certain accents in it nonetheless. A bay tree itself can be an accent, or you may want to add a sundial, a fountain or even a sculpture (as a nod to herb gardens of old) to add interest.

And just because it's informal and small doesn't mean it's without some type of structure. Think of the borders of your garden. You'll want something that grows low. And you'll want to probably keep it looking somewhat uniform. So you don't want to put three or five different plants along the border.

Maintain a constant border with one herb, perhaps parsley. You'd be surprised at how this pulls the entire concept of your garden together. If you want to use two or maybe even three plants as a border, arrange them in a way that you have a visually pleasing pattern to them.

Grouping your plants.

When deciding where exactly your specific herbs will live, you really don't have to worry about breaking any hard and fast gardener's rules. But it might help you if you separated those herbs that like the dry soil -- like the rosemary and thyme -- from those that need more moisture -- like basil and parsley.

And of course, place the herbs that you use most frequently as close to your kitchen door as possible. As much as we're aiming for beauty in the garden, the ultimate goal of this culinary herb garden is to enhance your cooking. If the garden isn't functional, then it's just not successful, no matter how beautiful it is.

Your private tea garden.

A garden dedicated to the growing of herbs just for tea is not a novel idea. And when the weather is nice, the garden is not only a source of your tea, but it can be the setting where you are able to leisurely sip your tea and meditate. It may also be the place to serve this fine beverage to your guests.

Let your imagination rule when it comes to the design of this specific garden. You can use any type of shape or configuration from an informal and cottage plan to a more formal approach or even a Zen like creation.

It's not unusual to walk into a backyard only to discover the tea garden the owners have created is in the shape of a teapot. Some individuals shape their gardens like teacups, complete with saucers.

Consider this fun idea: a teapot shaped garden, about eight to ten feet (two - three metres) from the lid to the bottom of the "pot." The size from handle on one end to the spout of the other would be about ten to twelve feet (three – three and half metres). This size is large enough to contain fifteen to twenty plants, all generously spaced.

Your only real limitation with this design is the sunlight available – and, of course, if your yard can accommodate such a design. Just bear in mind that (and I know this seems pretty darned obvious!), the larger the garden, the more maintenance it demands.

When creating your tea garden -- no matter what shape you ultimately decide it'll be -- keep in mind that historically they have been places for reflection and relaxation. You can create an addition sense of calm by generating a feeling of enclosure within this space.

Use hedges, trellises or even wooden fences to set this space apart. If you can't use any of these or don't like these ideas, why not enclose using rows of potted plants.

A Basic Guide to Growing Herbs

What is a tea garden without a tea table and a set of chairs or at least benches? Sit here alone, with family or a close friend to enjoy a cup of tea made from your own fresh herbs.

Accent your garden with tea-related "accessories."

Now here's a cute idea! Why not edge your garden bed with some old teaspoons or even mismatched saucers turned on end. You may even want to attach old teacups to garden stakes. Use these as plant markers.

Why not take your garden to the next level with accessorising? Buy a few used teapots at yard sales, swap meets, or thrift stores. Plant a few herbs in these to display in your garden. You can also plant a few herbs in a setting of teacups as well.

Beyond that you can use teacups as birdbaths as well. Actually if you set your imagination free, there's no end to how you can decorate your tea garden.

Whether you pay any attention to the design of your garden to create an elaborate back yard theme, or you decide to grow a few functional herbs from your windowsill or within handy access to your back door, you'll be taking that first exciting step to "communing" with nature as you've never known it before.

The aromatic fragrances of herbs are not only enticing, they're downright mesmerising. Add to that the beauty of some of the most stunning flowers Mother Nature ever made. Oh, yes. This is one addictive hobby.

Now let's get down to the real business of herb gardening: the herbs themselves.

Chapter Four:
Outdoor Gardening

In a nutshell, here's what it takes to grow healthy herbs outside. The right soil, just enough water (and not too much), and protection from the cold, winter months. And yes, one more thing: companion plants would help. Find out about all of these aspects of growing your herbs outdoors in this chapter.

It is one of those no-brainers. Healthy, vigorous herbs sprout from healthy, nutritious soil. Good soil is the basis of plants that are resistant to insect pests and various diseases. The pleasant surprise is that creating a healthy base for your herbs is incredibly easy.

Whether you're growing culinary, medicinal or tea herbs, they all need the same basic soil: three parts of garden soil, one part peat, compost or aged manure and one part sand. It's that easy. Give your herbs this and you're well on your way to producing healthy, strong herbs.

Beyond that you'll notice that many herbal guides advise the soil be "well drained." It's just a fact of herbal life -- these plants hate wet soil. You may be wondering how to ensure that the soil in your yard is well drained.

A Basic Guide to Growing Herbs

To build this ideal growing condition, simply place a three-inch layer of compressed stone into your soil about fifteen to eighteen inches (thirty-eight - forty-five cm) under the surface. Return the soil -- blended with compost and sand -- on top of these stones. Be sure in doing this, that you fill this topsoil just a little higher than it was originally. This allows for some settling of the soil as time passes.

As an additional insurance policy, you may also want to purchase a soil-moisture metre. Because this device actually measures the moisture at the roots of the plant, this can eliminate a lot of the guesswork that's usually involved in estimating moisture.

While you think the best, fastest and easiest way to obtain healthy plants is to fertilise them, and this is certainly true -- but just to an extent, just as with everything else in this world moderation is the key in nourishing your plants.

You may be surprised to learn that this is a point of diminishing returns when it comes to fertilising herbs. Herbs grown in overly fertilised soil actually grow poorly.

Your herbs aren't completely maintenance free. They require regular care and attention, just like flowers or vegetable plants. After the initial planting of the herbs, continue to apply compost or fertiliser to them on a regular basis. You may also want to add mulch occasionally as well. Mulch helps to preserve moisture. It also prevents weeds from overtaking your garden.

Many herb growers are concerned though with the plants they grow in containers. One of the questions I receive most often is how can you be certain your container herb is well drained. It really isn't as hard as it seems.

When you initially buy your pot or container for your plants, be sure the container already has drainer holes in it. The better containers will. If you decide to decorate, planting your herbs in unconventional containers -- say a teapot, for example -- then create several holes in the bottom to ensure proper drainage.

These holes don't need to be large. But to ease your worry that the soil will leak through these holes, fill the bottom of the container with gravel or stones. In this way, you'll be sure that the soil won't escape.

If you're planning on growing these herbs indoors, keep a waterproof tray underneath your pots. But be careful not to water these plants too much.

Specific soil for certain herbs.

Of course, one soil doesn't necessarily fit all herbs. There are different needs for different plants. And this is where the expertise of your local nursery is indispensible. They'll know exactly what type of soil your particular herbs need.

How often do my herbs like to drink?

Ahh! What a smart person you are to question this right up front. Obviously, you're either an accomplished experienced gardener ... or you were like me for the longest time -- killing off plants by either withholding water or drowning the poor things.

Here's a good rule of thumb that I've finally found works for me. When the natural rainfall is less than one inch within the week, water your herbs.

And don't forget that one of the very good uses for mulch is an effective control mechanism. When you go to the nursery to buy your mulch, be aware that you'll have a variety from which to choose.

Consider buying the bark chips or the shredded bark. Other good mulches you might consider include compost, ground corncobs, pecan hulls or even dried grass clippings.

When you spread your mulch, don't be cheap! You need to spread enough so that it has half a chance of performing the jobs you want it to. That means you want it at least three inches deep.

A Basic Guide to Growing Herbs

Surviving a cold, hard winter.

While it might not seem like a "Valley-Forge Experience" to you, the winter months may prove hard on your plants. You may want to take a bit of extra care when it comes to their winter protection and survival.

Granted, many of the perennial herbs are quite hardy. They survive the winter quite well, thank you. But depending on the other types of herbs you've planted outside and where you live, you may have to supply your plants with a little extra protection.

This is especially true if you live in any part of your country that gets rather extreme cold weather such as frost and snow. But more than just the cold, more herbs are killed by the extreme and wild fluctuations in temperature rather than just the extreme cold.

To make sure your herbs see it through to another summer, what you do throughout the growing season plays a vital role. I know I'm sounding like a broken record, but there's a reason I keep returning the theme of "well-drained" soil. It's just another layer of protection for your plant during the cold winter months.

If the soil herbs are sitting in isn't well drained they can be subjected to root rot over the winter months. So if you haven't

A Basic Guide to Growing Herbs

lightened up your soil throughout the summer months, come fall make it a priority. It's the best way to help ensure herbal survival in the winter.

Don't fertiliser or prune in winter.

You probably wouldn't do either of these, but I had to make myself clear on this point as well. Just as generally over-fertilising is not good, it's especially so once the winter months hit.

Pruning should only take place in the spring and summer months. When fall appears, you will be able to gradually pull back on your pruning. You actually will really want a little more growth in the fall; it helps to insulate the plants for the upcoming cold weather.

Also, considering protecting your herbs with an extra layer of mulch. Top the existing mulch off with evergreen branches or even some other material. Try not to use mulch that packs heavily down. It will only retain the moisture during the winter, which very well may contribute to root rot.

Got herbs that you feel are marginally hardy? Rosemary? Greek oregano? If you have doubts about their ability to survive the winter, then by all means don't be afraid to dig them up, pot them and bring them inside for the winter. Once spring hits, they can be planted outside again.

Diseases, insects and other pests.

Herbs grown outdoors and have access to ample air circulation, sunlight and water drainage are seldom affected with either disease or damage by insects.

The usual suspects that attack herbs -- mites and aphids -- are held in check by natural predators and parasites. And this is especially true if you're growing a wide variety of different herbs. Of course, you don't want to use chemical insecticides.

Instead, search out insecticidal soap as well as horticultural oil. These can help fight any attacks as well as keeping your plants chemical free! If you have troubles with some of the larger pests, like beetles and caterpillars, you can just simply pick them off.

Companion plants.

Sounds like a buddy movie aimed at wildlife. But when it comes to herbs, companion plants may prove to be a vital key in the overall health of your garden -- not only your herb garden, but your patch of vegetables and your flowerbed too!

That's because some plants actually grow better when they're sitting next to other plants. Now, it might not sound very sensible, but the concept really is very simple.

A Basic Guide to Growing Herbs

When you begin to add specific herbs to either your vegetable or flower garden -- or both -- you will notice a decidedly improved level of overall health for all the plants, depending on the herbs you've put there.

Let me give you a classic example of this. And when I say classic, I'm drawing on history. When white settlers arrived in North America, they soon learned that the Native Americans had what they referred to as the "three Sisters" a combination of corns, beans and squash. Now if you learned this in school or elsewhere as I did, you might have assumed these three plants were "sisters" because they were a vital part of their overall diet. And that's true!

But here's the rest of the story. When planted together, they actually help the others to grow. The beans, first of all are the "nitrogen-fixers" for the other plants and they climb the stalks of the corn. The squash shades the ground for the sake of the health of the other two plants holding the moisture longer in the ground.

More examples of companion plants.

Now, here's an example that might have come straight from your garden. Garlic and roses. As much as it might sound like a new heavy metal rock band, it's really how many gardeners arrange their plants. Having garlic and roses together is companion planting.

A Basic Guide to Growing Herbs

The pungent scent of the garlic repels a portion of the rose plant's worst pests, the aphids. Cool isn't it? Actually to a gardener who is really trying to stay organic, it's quite thrilling.

But you also have the opposite affect. Some plants just don't grow well at all when placed together. Did you know that Irish potatoes don't grow well at all when placed next to turnips or pumpkins?

While I may sound as if I'm not taking this very seriously, there's actually very good reasons for these companion plants -- or in this case, non-companion plants. Tall plants may block the sun from lower lying sun-loving plants. Others may actually create some negative biochemical reaction with those around them.

Here are a few other herbs you may want to consider planting with others - as well as some you may want to keep these herbs from getting near.

Basil. This plant adores tomatoes. And they really are brilliant together, not only in the garden, but on the plate too. In fact they are so good together some gardeners have developed a rule of (green) thumb: three basil plants for every tomato plant.

But here's one more thing you may not have known about basil -- it actually repels flies and mosquitoes.

A Basic Guide to Growing Herbs

Borage. This particular herb encourages the growth of strawberries. It also goes well with tomatoes and squash.

Chamomile. Be sure to plant these with your onions and cabbage -- and watch all three of them grow strong and healthy.

Chives. Did you know that if you steep chives in water, it's an ingenious way of killing powdery mildew disease organically? And when you plant it, you'll want it near your carrots if you have a vegetable garden and any apple trees you may have on your property.

Dill. Dill appreciates being near corn, cabbage, lettuce, and cucumbers. However, don't plant dill near fennel just to avoid cross-pollination.

Garlic. Of course, we've already mentioned how this plant loves tomatoes, but you can also plant it near fruit trees as well. Garlic repels the red spider mites. And this herb, steeped in water is another effective insecticide.

Lemon balm. Plant this plant with the tomatoes.

Mint. It'll help cabbage grow, but don't let it get near your parsley.

A Basic Guide to Growing Herbs

Oregano. Think collard, broccoli, cauliflower, and cabbage. And then plant the oregano plant with these.

Parsley. You'll make your parsley and your tomato plants both happy if you companion plant them. You can also plant parsley with carrots, chives and even asparagus. But keep the parsley away from the mint.

Rosemary. Keep her away from the potatoes. But, you'll want to plant this herb near cabbage, carrots, beans and sage, go ahead.

Sage. In addition to rosemary, sage also encourages the growth and health of carrots, and cabbage. But please keep it away from your cucumber.

Thyme. Cabbage appreciates being near thyme. The added benefit is that this herb wards off worms that love to chomp on the cabbage.

Now that you know how to keep your outside herbs healthy and happy, let's see what it takes to maintain quality herbs inside your home. That's the focus of the next chapter.

A Basic Guide to Growing Herbs

Chapter Five:
Indoor Gardening

While growing herbs indoors is very handy indeed, it does depend on a large part on the delicate balance of soil, water and light. Discover just how crucial these three elements are.

Gardening outdoors sounds great, doesn't it? But a bit more than you're willing to handle right now? I can totally understand that. If the lure of the fresh herbs is whispering your name, but your back is screaming enough already, then perhaps you should consider confining your initial foray into herbs to your home.

Actually, there are some advantages to this, not the least of which is growing a small group of herbs -- and maintaining their health. Your taste buds will thank you, the herbs of courses will thank you and your back will be grateful as well.

Perhaps you would rather start small - and indoors. Many people do. Many discover their love of herbs after they've grown several merely for practical purposes, never suspecting they would end up with a life long love of the plants.

If that's the case your kitchen herb garden may very well take the form of a window box full of plants or perhaps just a group of planters in your kitchen. However, don't just throw this together without some basic forethought even if it is only a small widow box.

I see the light!

There's really only one catch to growing herbs -- especially in the initial stages. These plants crave -- and they really do need! -- ten to twelve hours of sunlight every day to thrive. And herbs really do prefer natural light to artificial light.

Before you make your final decision on what herbs to grow, you will need to work out exactly the amount of sunlight that comes through your kitchen windows. This will ultimately dictate which herbs you *can* grow.

If your windowsills aren't wide enough to place containers on them, consider extending the sills. No you don't have to be a carpenter to do this. It is a simple as adding a finished slim board to the windowsill. Just screw it into the existing board of the sill. If you just can't bring yourself to place screws in your sills, I understand.

Or you may want to consider looking purchasing one of the windowsill extenders that cat lovers use to ensure their felines have a nice view of the outdoors. You should be able to get several plants on one of these.

Your local hardware store will be able to advise you.

A Basic Guide to Growing Herbs

But if you don't want to do that, simply put shelving up in front of the window.

The only step left is to figure out which specific windows face which direction. This you'll need to know as an avid indoor gardener. You can easily Google which side of your home (North, South East, West) in your country are privy to the longest lasting and the brightest light.

This also means that this is the hottest portion of your home. However, there will be some herbs that won't want to live there. The more tender of your plants may burn with that much light.

So have them on the sill of the more indirect light and much less heat coming through the windows of your house. Light on the other two sides offer bright light, but there's really nothing that can compare with that sunny exposure.

And yes, you really should turn your plants once a week or so to allow the sunlight to reach all sides of the plant.

Artificial light.

If even on your best windows you can't give them that, then perhaps you should invest in a grow light. This form of lighting is relatively inexpensive and you can find them at just about nursery or discount stores and even hardware stores.

You'll want the artificial lights to be about ten inches (twenty-five cm) above the young herb starters. For more mature or larger plants, hang them about a foot to a foot and a half (thirty to forty-five cm) above the plants.

And yes, keep these lights on the plants about ten hours a day. This simulates the time the sun would be shining on these guys.

Let there be light! But what kind of light?

Talk to any three cultivators of indoor herbs and you're very likely to receive three very distinct and opinionated ideas when it comes to what kind of light to place above your herbs. You have basically two choices: fluorescent and high-intensity discharge light.

Let's talk about fluorescent lighting first. This kind is the most recognisable to us: you see them everywhere. They're usually long and thin. And believe it or not, home gardeners have used this specific type of lighting for years. It's especially useful for starting seeds. But it's also good at encouraging growth in plants as well.

The intensity of the fluorescent light is low, so they really are ideal for encouraging the growth of seedlings. But these are also ideal for low-growing herbs. Even the lowest leaves are close to the light with these.

Consider this: a standard four-foot (one hundred and twenty cm) unit with two forty-watt bulbs -- or tubes -- illuminates an area of about eight inches (20 cm) in width.

But more than that, you can also buy specialty tubes for your specific needs. There are an array of tubes are available, depending on the needs of your herbs.

But don't overlook a combination of the standard cool and warm white tubes. These seem to be effective. Verilux tubes are another choice. This type of light is the closest approximation to the sun, so experts say. (I personally have to take their word for it!).

On the other hand, a brand called Vita-Lite, is labelled as a "power twist" tube. It produces somewhat more light than the standard fluorescent does per watt. And the quality of this light is well balanced for optimum plant growth.

The brightness of light is measured either in lumens or as foot candles. Lumens is a reference to the amount of light available at the source. Foot candles measures the amount of light falling on the area. As you move farther from the light, then, the lumens would naturally stay the same. However, as you can imagine, the farther you travelled from the light, the amount of foot candles would decrease.

A Basic Guide to Growing Herbs

A bright but overcast day measures about one thousand foot candles. By contrast, a bright sunshiny day generates about ten thousand foot candles. I don't mention this randomly either.

Contrast this to fluorescent lights. You'll be receiving about seven hundred foot candles when the herbs are six inches from the source. A foot from the light, the foot-candle measurement drops to forty-five hundred.

What about humidity?

The ultimate dry environment of your house may present another problem in growing your plants indoors. If you don't have a complete humidifier system through your home (I certainly don't!), you will be able to provide the perfect humidity for these plants at a cost that is easy on the budget.

First, remember to finely mist the plants with water on a weekly basis. I did say this wasn't going to cost you an arm and a leg! You can also add humidity to the specific area where the plants are simply by setting a dish of water near the heat source in the room. As the heat source is operating, it will naturally evaporate the water, which adds moisture into the air.

Another good way to moisturise the plants is to fill trays with pea gravel. Additionally, pour water into these trays so the

A Basic Guide to Growing Herbs

water fills about half the tray. Now simply set the plants on top of the gravel.

Any one of these -- or using all three of these in extreme measures! -- should solve even the toughest of the humidity problems.

How much water do these plants like?

That's a good question. Herbs grown in containers do tend to dry out more quickly than those grown outside. But there's not need for concern as it's easy enough to check the status. Simply stick a finger into the soil. Make sure you get at least get half an inch below the surface to feel the moisture.

If the soil feels dry to the touch, then you'll need to water the plant some. As much as you may be tempted, don't overwater these indoor herbs. You'll only be promoting root rot as well as the development of a disease called powdery mildew.

This plant disease is probably one of the most . If your herb is afflicted with this, it would look as if it had powdery splotches of white or gray on not only the leaves, but also on its stems.

While this disease is not fatal, it does indeed stress the plant. In fact, repeated infections will weaken the plant. And if the mildew is not corrected, it may cover so much of the plant it eventually cripples the plants ability to go through photosynthesis.

The case of Powdery Mildew.

Should one of your herbs become infected with powdery mildew, caring for it is much easier than you may think. Your first move of course is to remove and destroy all areas that are infected.

You'll then want to improve the circulation of your plants. And no you don't do this by making it run a marathon or putting it on a treadmill! Thin your plants out and prune the affected plants.

While the herb is infected don't fertilise it. You may find that a bit contradictory because I've just said this mildew weakens the plant. But the disease thrives on young, succulent growth. So while you and your herb are actually battling this problem, refrain from fertilising it.

And another tip on trying to discourage the mildew: don't water the plants from above. When you water the plants, move the lowest branches around in order to pour the water straight on the soil itself. You really don't want to get the stems wet.

You may be forced eventually to apply a fungicide to some of your herbs. Now that doesn't mean you're using harsh

A Basic Guide to Growing Herbs

chemicals. That would certainly negate some of the reasons for growing these specific plants at home.

No, the fungicide you'll be applying -- and you can simply ask any nursery about this -- is created from such natural ingredients as potassium bicarbonate, sulphur or even copper.

Now let's talk the actual planting!

It's about time, you're probably thinking. But, it's important to know what to do with your plants. Now you'll learn how to plant them properly. Taking care of them during the growing season will now be a breeze -- or at least easier than you may have imagined when you first started.

Believe it or not, you're pretty well set already. If you're starting with nothing (as many first-time gardeners are) you'll want to ensure that you have a good supply of six-inch (fifteen cm) planting pots. This is probably the best size herb pot.

You can grow many seeds or small bulbs in just one of these pots, adhering to the "one-inch apart" dogma with the bulbs. (You'll recall that all bulbs need to be at least one inch (two and half cm) apart in order to grow healthy.)

Before you place any kind of soil -- or combination of media -- into these pots, line them with stones and bark chips. This serves as your drainage system as well as an effective aeration mechanism.

When you do fill these pots, don't use just any soil. (Herbs are a bit in the "snobbish, elite" range when it comes to that!). Use a good quality soil. It should be loose as well as containing as many of the nutrients as possible that your plants will need. Your nursery will tell you the right soil for herbs.

Bury these seeds or small bulbs in the pots about an inch (two and half cm) apart across the entire surface of the container.

If, on the other hand, you're transplanting nursery-bought seedlings you have two choices. First, you can remove these plants from their original containers, placing them in the holes you've dug into the potting soil. The other option is to plant them and their containers in the potting soil together.

While this second selection may sound a bit off the wall, it has a definite advantage. When planting the container with the herb, you are assured that the plant has its root systems intact and undamaged. It also just happens to make growing and transplanting several herbs much quicker and easier.

It's also easy to recognise when you the herbs have outgrown their homes. A plant can grow in the same pot for one season.

The telltale sign that it needs transplanted? Its roots are beginning to burst out of its container. Don't worry about taking it out of that container. Just follow the same steps as you have previously. The plant will thrive, trust me!

Chapter Six:
Caring for the Herbs.

Planting, transplanting, starting your herbs from seeds, harvesting and preserving. Once you get your plants growing, you'll no doubt want to keep them from year to year -- somehow. This chapter shows you how. This chapter also gives you some tips on harvesting and preserving your herbs for the off-season.

Yes, the growing season has been lovely. But there is a time when it just has to come to an end. And it looks like fall is fast approaching. It feels as if winter is just around the corner. So what does a good herb gardener do right about now?

No, you don't sit down and cry, lamenting about a lost season. This is the time you can spring into action, harvesting the herbs you have, preserving them for the long winter -- and transplanting those you can to keep them growing next year as well.

It may sound like work, but keep in mind that these herbs have provided you with an incredible amount of joy this spring and summer. And they're about to provide you with more flavourful meals during the cold winter months. And some of these herbs may just help you avoid some of the toughest germs, and colds going around this winter.

A Basic Guide to Growing Herbs

Besides, you know darn well this really isn't work -- it's a labour of love.

If you're planting or even transplanting seedlings outside, the best method I've found is to dig the hole, adding just a "dash" of compost and bone meal for drainage as well as extra nutrients.

You'll discover as you grow a larger variety of herbs that many herbs grow best in an alkaline soil. Knowing this, you may want to add a tablespoon or two of agricultural lime. This helps the roots to absorb nutrients more efficiently. All of this gets mixed into the soil in the hole before putting the herb in.

You'll discover too that even though your herbs are eventually destined to be part of an outdoor garden, you'll want to start them indoors. Some herbs just seem to get a much healthier start when begun inside. Some of the plants you may want to start inside include basil, borage, marjoram, oregano, chamomile, catnip, sorrel and thyme.

Simply place the seeds in the pots containing well-drained, airy soil with lots of organic matter. Borage and sorrel, though, would rather be in soil that is moist and rich.

When your seedlings are about four inches (ten cm) tall and the weather is warm, you're ready to "introduce" them to the outside environment. As strange as this may sound, it is very necessary. It's a step many beginning gardeners just don't do, simply because they are unaware that they have to.

Introducing these plants gradually to the out of doors is called hardening off. This process should not be intense until the overnight temperatures rise to a dependable fifty degrees F (ten degrees C) or more.

Also, ensure that the plants you're "hardening off" are placed in sturdy containers with moist soil. Start the process simply by placing the pots outside starting at nine a.m. Leave them here for several hours.

Remember that you are dealing with delicate seedlings. Don't take them out on windy days. These guys are small; even a light gust may knock the pots off the deck or patio.

The potential for broken stems in this situation is extremely real. If any of your plants, by the way have any lids or cellophane coverings, by all means remove them before you take them out. On the first day be especially vigilante that the soil doesn't dry out or the leaves don't droop.

Repeat this process for the next five or six days. Every day increase the amount of time the seedlings spend outdoors. The only exception to this is the unexpected, wild fluctuations of temperature as sometimes happen during the spring.

A Basic Guide to Growing Herbs

If the temperature varies more than fifteen degrees from one day to the next in either direction -- warmer or colder -- then shorten the seedlings exposure outside. Basically, what you're doing is acclimatizing your plants to the environment.

Don't place the herbs out if it is extremely rainy or excessively hot. The process won't be ruined when they're kept in for a day or so.

Do this for about five days. After that your plants should be ready to be planted outdoors.

Alternatives to hardening off.

Some herbalists prefer to use other methods than the hardening off to prepare the seedlings for the outdoor garden. One method is a low-water approach.

In this method, you don't place the plants outside, you leave them indoors, but you decrease the watering of them in increments. Each time, allow the soil to dry out a little more than the last time. Do this for two to three weeks.

Eventually you'll only water them when they begin to droop. Once they're to this point, they're ready for the outside world.

A Basic Guide to Growing Herbs

Propagating new plants.

You've planted your herbs, they all seem to be doing quite nicely thank you. But now, you'd really like to take that next step. Propagating new plants.

There are three main methods you can do this. You can create more plants through dividing the roots of the existing plants, by taking cuttings of the herbs in your gardens or through a method called healing in or layering.

Root division.

This is a simple approach to creating more herbs. With a spade or shovel, work the roots from a clump of the densely growing herbs. Taking this grouping out of the ground, separate the plants starting at the roots. You want to do this rather carefully.

Once separated you can place one of the groupings back in the original spot. The other group or groups may be planted anywhere you like.

Creating herbs from cuttings.

This is another straightforward approach to propagating herbs. In either the spring or the fall, you'll take a long, woody shoot

A Basic Guide to Growing Herbs

from the plant of your choosing. Cut the shoot at an angle close the ground.

Remove the leaves from the very bottom of this cutting. Coating it with a rooting powder, you'll pot it in a light soil mix. Water this well.

Creating new herbs through layering.

Bend a long woody shoot; bury the middle of the stem under a few inches of soil. Hold it down with a small rock. Within a month to six weeks, the cutting or the healed-in stem develops its own root system. It's at this time that it's ready to be transplanted.

Harvesting, preserving herbs.

Growing herbs is just part of the fun of keeping your herb garden. Though I have to admit it's a great deal of fun. Another aspect of herb gardening which many people enjoy is the harvesting and the preserving of the herbs once the growing season ends.

Ask five different herb gardeners and you're bound to get five different ideas about the best method to harvest these plants. The great herbalist and nun of the twelfth Century, Hildegard of Bingen firmly believed that all medicinal plants should be harvested when the moon is waxing, that is, just prior to it

A Basic Guide to Growing Herbs

becoming full. When herbs are taken at this time, she believed they possessed their greatest potency.

She did concede, though, that the herbs would be preserved for an extended period of time if they were harvested during the waning of the moon.

Many herbalists have other ideas though. Many believe, for instance that herbs should be gathered only during a full moon. This is the time, they say, when the sap and the strength of their oils are the greatest.

While you may consider these ideas "old wives' tales" they do seem to have a bit of validity. The time of harvesting seem to play a part in the potency.

Herbs whose medicinal active ingredients are found in their roots and rhizomes -- like ginger, ginseng and mandrake, for instance -- are more potent when harvested in late autumn or in early spring. At this time, they have actually retained much of their energy and essence below the ground.

When you harvest this type of herb, you want to dig widely around the plants, so you don't cut or damage the root system. Use cold water to wash the roots and thoroughly dry them.

It's also true the essence of a plant becomes concentrated with each subsequent night. Therefore, the herbs are most potent when they're picked in the early hours of the morning well before the sun's heat and the light actually dissipate any essential oils in them.

And it's best to harvest the herbs on a morning that is clear and dry, as soon as the dew has evaporated from the leaves. Nearly all herbs should be harvesting before they bloom.

The active healing substances of these plants also lose their potency after the flowering process, for obvious reasons. They've just spent much of their energy on actually blooming and generating seeds.

When you do harvest herbs, be sure to use a good pair of sharp pruning clippers, as you don't want to tear the stems. As long as you don't cut down too low on the stem, you'll discover that some herbs -- basil is particularly noted for this -- will produce more growth for harvest.

As a part of keeping your garden growing, you may decide to deliberately *not harvest* several plants of various species. You may decide to allow them to seed towards the growth of next year's garden.

These seeds are really easy to collect. The best idea is to pre-determine which plants you want to go to seed. Just before the seeds mature, you need to place a paper bag over each flower,

A Basic Guide to Growing Herbs

upside down. With a bit of string or twine, tie the mouth of the bag so it is snug.

Once the seeds have matures, you need to cut off each seed head keeping the bag attached. Then, turn the bag so it is the right way up, tap the seeds so they fall into the bag then remove the string and you have a bag full of seeds.

Preserving your herbs.

I admit, my initial idea of preserving herbs was taking the bottle of ginseng and placing it in a cool, dry place, just like the label instructed. Guess what? I soon discovered fresh herbs didn't work that way.

What I did learn that preserving and storing fresh herbs is every bit as fun and rewarding as growing them. And this is especially true when it comes to medicinal herbs.

And don't worry, I promise you this process is neither difficult nor painful on your part.

Now that you've harvested the herbs, you'll want them to last as long as possible. The drying process is the best way to achieve this. In days past, it was custom to simply hang the herbs in a warm, dry, shady location, waited until they crumbled easily and placed them in various containers.

Custom also dictated that the roots were washed, split and then spread into a single layer on a clean tray. And this method is still practiced diligently by a few herbalists. It isn't unusual to walk into a herb shop and actually buy a "bunch" of herbs.

But, that's not to say it's the best approach. In fact, there are two distinct disadvantages to using this method. First, it takes up a lot of space, sometimes more space than you can devote.

The other disadvantage is the time factor. Yes, it takes at a minimum a few days, and in some instances weeks for the leaves, stems and flowers to dry on their own. And we haven't even begun to talk about the roots, which in some instances may take up to a month or more to completely dry properly.

Time is of the essence, literally!

When drying herbs for medicinal or healing purposes, time is literally of the essence. The faster the herbs are dried, the more potent the volatile aromatic oils in the herbs will be. And that's precisely why most of the commercial herb producers use special equipment for drying herbs.

In order to speed the process somewhat many herb gardeners simply place their herbs on a baking sheet or on a section of clean window screen, then place this is an oven set at ninety-five degrees F (thirty-five degrees C).

This method is not only convenient, but inexpensive as well. Of course, this has a few disadvantages. One of the biggest being that in the heat of summer not many people really want to use the oven to cook -- let alone for drying herbs.

If your oven, moreover, is one of those (and there are many out there) that don't heat evenly, it can cause you some problems. Some of the herbs may actually dry out too much, while other sections are too moist.

Now, you say, I'm knocking down options right and left. So what's left? Some herbalists buy a small produce dryer. This is a tabletop appliance with built-in removable trays. It uses a hot air fan to dry the herbs. As you might have already guessed by its name, it also dries produce.

Drying is just the beginning.

Whoa! Don't stop now! Drying is just the first step in the preservation process. Once the herbs have dried, many herbalists then reduce them to a powder. This is the most convenient form for use.

Traditionally, herbalists have made their powders using the old-fashioned mortar and pestle. And it's a method that many still use today, especially if you don't have many herbs to grind.

If that seems a bit old fashioned to you -- as it did to me -- try grinding your herbs in a coffee grinder. You may want to

A Basic Guide to Growing Herbs

purchase one separately for this purpose. You might not want the flavours of either mixing with the other.

Coffee-flavoured lemon balm is just as bad as basil-flavoured coffee. I find it far easier to have a separate grinder for the herbs rather than use the same one for both herbs and coffee, however the choice is yours.

For those gardeners who have large amounts of herbs, a large grinder is advisable.

Storing your herbs.

Take a quick look at the bottled commercially bought herbs and spices you already have in your kitchen cabinet, please. Carefully examine the bottle they're in. Is it a clear glass or plastic bottle?

Chances are it is clear. That way you can actually see the type of spice you're purchasing. At least that's my take on why the bottles are clear. And probably because clear bottles may cost less than dark amber ones.

But you're about to learn a powerful lesson in preserving herbs: clear glass is the worst thing you can keep your dried herbs in. And here's why: light may be the giver of life for these plants for so long, but it is also the destroyer of potency and flavour once the herbs are dry. It's ironic, but it's true.

A Basic Guide to Growing Herbs

Instead, store your dried herbs in opaque containers -- glass or ceramic are the best ones to use. Fill the container to the top. This limits the amount of oxygen in them. As you use your herbs and there are less of them in the container, you can prevent oxygen from getting inside by adding cotton to the jar.

Carefully stored aromatic herbs, like rosemary, thyme and sage, are actually able to remain potent for a year and more. Herbs that don't carry much of a fragrance, like alfalfa, will last longer.

Moisture kills.

Moisture is another enemy of your dried herbs. If they do happen to get wet once they've been dried, try and get them quickly dried again. This will prevent the growth of mould.

You'll also want to be vigilant to the problem of insects. Drying takes care of many different pests, but always keep your eyes open for insects. If you keep the containers tightly closed when you're not actually using the herbs, it will help to avoid this problem.

Freezing fresh herbs.

So far, we've discussed drying herbs to use later -- especially if these are for healing purposes. However, there's no reason why you can't freeze culinary herbs. This is very simple to do and

A Basic Guide to Growing Herbs

makes cooking with them easy when you could use some "fresh" herbs for those soups in the winter.

This is all you do. Cut the stems or the leaves of the herbs then rinse them. After patting them dry, you can freeze them in re-sealable bags. The bags can be of the smaller variety, then you can take one bag out and have just enough for your meal.

You can also freeze chopped fresh herbs in ice cube trays with water. Transfer them into freezer bags once the water and herbs have frozen. This is the best way to use them for soup.

Now that autumn is approaching, you've harvested and preserved your herbs, what's left to do?

Why don't you just sit down with the cup of herbal tea and plan next season's garden.

Chapter Seven:
Preparing Herbal Remedies.

Are you ready? As you prepare your home-grown herbs to be used as remedies, remember that you are continuing a tradition that's as old as mankind himself. It's exciting -- and quite humbling -- to be part of a heritage that actually goes back to the Stone Age.

Herbs can be used to heal in a variety of ways. Here's how you heal yourself, your family and your friends by using a tincture-based herb.

A tincture is a preserved form of the herb, using some form of alcohol as the preservative. But more than that the alcohol is used to extract the active properties of the herb as well as concentrate them to ensure their effectiveness.

A tincture also has the advantage of being very easy for your body to use. Tinctures are indeed both concentrated and cost-effective.

There is one downside to them, however. When you drink a tincture, you receive the full flavour of the herb. And for some people this taste will be just too much. Some people may find this just downright unpleasant. Cayenne for example, will come through hot! And goldenseal, when used in a tincture has an extremely bitter taste.

Of course, the presence of the alcohol in this form of herbal preparation may bother right from the start. Quite frankly, I don't blame you one bit if it does. This is of special concern many times for parents. They would love to give their children a serving of the tincture herb to make them feel better, but they're fearful of the alcohol content of it. Some herbalists say that you can just lessen the concentration of the alcohol in the tincture by mixing the serving with one-quarter cup of very hot water.

Wait about five minutes, and then most of that alcohol taste will have evaporated. And the tincture should be cool enough to drink.

Making your own tincture.

You will need:
- Dried or fresh herbs
- Eighty to one hundred proof vodka or rum (Never use rubbing alcohol, also known as isopropyl alcohol or wood alcohol)
- Wide-mouth glass jar with lid (a canning jar is perfect)
- Unbleached cheesecloth or muslin
- Labels
- Markers
- Small amber glass bottles

Tincture Recipe.

The exact amount of the individual herb you use is up to you, depending on the amount of tincture you want on hand. A good rule of thumb is to use one part herb to every five parts of alcohol. It really doesn't matter how large that "part" is.

Place your herbs -- finely chopped -- into the canning jar. Pour the alcohol in the ratio advised into the jar. Make sure the alcohol base completely covers your herb.

Now close the lid tightly. Allow the herbs to soak for up to six weeks. During this time visit the jar every several days to shake it. The alcohol siphons and extracts the active ingredients from the herbs during this period.

At the end of six weeks, use a large sieve, strainer or other type of press to strain the mixture. Immediately take the wet herbs, wrapping them in muslin, cheesecloth or another type of fine cloth. Tightly but gently squeeze the herbs to get as much of the alcohol-based mixture off the herbs as possible.

The herbs that are the most saturated will naturally also be those that are strongest when it comes to carrying the active medicinal ingredients of healing power.

Your next step is take the herbs from your large container and place them in smaller glass bottles. Preferably, the bottles should be amber colour.

That's it! You've made your first tincture from your own herbs grown in your own garden. How clever and resourceful are you!

Oh, and by the by the way. The tincture you made today? It'll be effective for up to five years! That's what I'm talkin' about!

Herbal Plasters.

Okay, so the first time I heard this phrase I thought it meant a cast of some sort. I admit it. But nothing can be farther from the truth. It actually has little to do with plaster in any sense that you may be thinking about. And no, I really don't know why it's called a plaster.

But, a plaster is a thick, moist herbal paste that's warmed and placed between two layers of cheesecloth or muslin. Some herbalists use a cloth pouch. This is then placed directly on the skin where the irritation is. The herb itself, because it is wrapped in the cloth never actually touches the skin. And for this reason you need to be very careful in using one of these.

Most frequently used in the treatment of respiratory congestion, a plaster can also be used for such conditions as skin infections, irritable bowel syndrome and even high blood pressure.

A Basic Guide to Growing Herbs

Plasters work well because they release their oils which contain the healing ingredients.

When making a plaster, your first step is to grind your herb -- preferably a dried herb -- *immediately prior* to actually preparing the remedy itself. The grinding of the herb releases the pockets of enzymes which in turn active the essential oils of the plant.

Once you've ground your home-grown herbs, you then mix about quarter cup of the herb in just enough water lukewarm (never hot for this preparation) to make a thick paste-like concoction. Do not get this mixture in your eyes or under your fingernails.

Take this paste-like mixture, place it between several layers of clean cloth, like cheesecloth or muslin. Place the plaster over the affected area of the body.

After about five minutes, you'll notice a burning sensation. Don't be alarmed; this is part of the healing process. It's merely a signal that the herbal oils are penetrating the deeper layers of your skin.

Once this burning sensation begins though, you should remove the herbal plaster immediately. You have a window of about five to fifteen minutes when it can safely stay on your body. But fifteen minutes is really the very maximum.

A Basic Guide to Growing Herbs

A word of caution: if you have a circulatory problem, herbalist and nutritionists, Phyllis Balch advises in her book Prescriptions for Herbal Healing. Not to use a plaster for any reason.

Poultices.

A what? That might be your question when someone mentions the word, poultice. But an herbal poultice is nothing more than a thick, moist, warm herbal paste applied directly to the skin.

Its purpose is to relieve pain, inflammation as well as swelling or muscle spasms. You make poultices with your home-grown herbs, either while they are still fresh or after you've dried them.

To create a healing poultice from dried herbs, place a steamer, heat-proof colander, a strainer or even a sieve over a pot of rapidly boiling water. Place up to a quarter cup of your herb in the container. Reduce the heat under the water so it just simmers. Cover the pot.

Allow the steam to penetrate through the herbs until they are wilted. This should occur within five minutes. Then spread the softened, warmed herbs on cheesecloth, folding one layer of the cloth over the herb itself.

Apply this directly the affected area of your body. If you wish you can cover the poultice with a towel or even a woollen cloth. This will help it to retain the heat longer.

The poultice can remain in place for at least twenty minutes. In fact, you may even leave it on overnight. But it absolutely must be covered.

If you prefer to make your pulped poultice from fresh herbs, place the herbs between two layers of cheesecloth that's twice the size of the area affected. Take a rolling pin -- other equally heavy round object -- and finely crush the herbs. You'll know that the herbs are sufficiently crushed when the cloth feels damp from the moisture of the herbs themselves.

If you have a food processor, you may want to place the herbs in that. If you do this, then mix a small amount of hot water with them.

Now place a towel or woollen cloth over this to retain the "juices" and to help to hold the herbs in place. A poultice like this may also remain on the affected area overnight, if necessary.

The key to a poultice's effectiveness is that you use these particular set of herbs only once. Don't try to store a used poultice and use it again. Toss it and start all over again the following day or even several hours later.

A Basic Guide to Growing Herbs

I would suggest you use Google to find out just which herbs to use for the different ailments and whether it should be done as a tincture, a plaster or poultice.

Chapter Eight:
14 Tips To Help You Get Started

1. Seasonal plants: Decide if you want Perennial - plants that come back every single year, note that these may look as if they have died, but the roots are still alive so water them once or twice during the winter and they will sprout new growth in spring. - or Annuals - herbs that you will need to plant each year. You can also get self-seeing Annuals - plants that make their own seeds after flowering each year and may even replant themselves in the same spot if you let them go to seed.
2. Tag your herbs: Name each of the herbs until you get to know them otherwise you may be scratching your head trying to remember.
3. Sun: Remember to check if your herb needs sun, partial, sun, partial shade or no sun at all.
4. Water: If you keep the care tag you'll be able to check how often to water the plant. It will also tell you if the soil should be moist or not.
5. Height: Check how high the herb will grow and plant it in the garden accordingly.
6. Temperature: Herbs are amazingly resilient and can often continue growing even after a frost. Check on the care tag as it should say there what temperature it will be okay in.
7. Zones: Check the internet for your zone for growing.
8. Soil choices: Don't forget if you're planting outside that you

A Basic Guide to Growing Herbs

may need to amend the soil with compost and/or peat moss.

9. Check your tools: Make sure you have everything you need before you head off to plant your herbs regardless if it's the garden or the pots.
10. Take advice: Always have a talk to the nurseryman about which herbs are going to be best for your area and the time of year.
11. Companion planting: Read up about which plants go with which. This will definitely help your herbs to thrive (and vegetables too if you're planting in amongst your vegetable patch.)
12. Space: Make sure you plant your herbs out in such a way to give them space to grow. The care tag should give an indication of measurement required.
13. Drainage: Remember to make sure you have good drainage.
14. Be prepared for pests: You will need to decide if you want to be organic (recommended) or if you don't mind spraying. Just remember that if you do spray with chemicals you can easily be killing of the good insects as well as the uninvited!
15. Your best friend: Your nurseryman is definitely your best friend. They can help you with any gardening problem you may have from what to plant to where in the world you are and what will be best. The other friend you have is Google. For the kitchen and the culinary side, search the Internet for dishes that are using the herbs you are growing. For

example, Google 'recipes with basil' and you'll be surprised just how many options will come up. The same can be done for the healing plants and how to use them.

Most of all ... Enjoy!

A Basic Guide to Growing Herbs

Conclusion.

It really wasn't as difficult as you envisioned it at first, now was it? When approached properly, herbal gardening is one of the joys of nature. It's relaxing to do -- and provides hours on hours of potential peace and serenity in the growing season.

From basil to chives to sage and thyme, each herb has its own special characteristics, special growing quirks and its specialties on your kitchen table and for healing your body. Each herb, you've discovered, has in effect its own "personality."

I certainly hope you've enjoyed learning about herbs as much as I've enjoyed writing about them. Hopefully, you'll continue on with your new hobby -- I can't see why you wouldn't -- and discover even more about herbs next growing season.

There's always something to learn. After more years than I care to admit growing these fantastic plants, I'm still learning something new everyday about the proper way to water them, harvest them, store them ... or any number of things.

Don't become discouraged if some of your plants fizzled out this year. Certainly don't believe that your thumb isn't green enough to be an herb gardener. It happens to the best of us. It still happens to me to this day.

A certain percentage of herbs just don't seem to make it sometimes. Sometimes we know why -- we've had an extremely rainy summer or we didn't provide for enough drainage. Sometimes though these things just happen -- and leave even the best of gardeners scratching their heads in wonder.

Well, this is where I leave you. But, thankfully you're now surrounded by your herbs. Take care -- and take care of your garden.

Happy Gardening!
Fee

Appendix I:
What Your Herbs need.

Growing Requirements, Propagation and Uses of Herbs

ANNUAL HERBS.

Anise. *Pimpinella anisum:*

grows twenty-four inches (sixty to sixty-five cm) needs ten inches (twenty-five cm) space when planting needs full sun. Can be propagated from seed

Uses: Put leaves into soups, sauces, and salads; oil for flavoring; seeds for seasoning breads, cookies and cakes

Basil, sweet. *Ocimum basilicum:*

grows twenty-twenty-four inches (sixty to sixty-five cm) needs six –twelve inches (fifteen - thirty cm) space when planting, needs full sun. Can be propagated from seed, grow transplants for early-season harvest.

Uses: Put leaves into soups, stews, pasta sauce, poultry and meat dishes; flavors vinegar; teas.

Borage. *Borago officinalis:*

grows one – three feet (thirty - ninety cm) needs twelve inches (thirty cm) space when planting, needs full sun. Can be propagated from seed, self-sowing.

Uses: Edible flower; leaves in salads, teas, and sandwiches; attracts bees.

Calendula (Pot Marigold). *Calendula officinalis*:

grows twelve inches (thirty cm) needs twelve – eighteen inches (30 – 45 cm) space when planting, needs sun, partial shade. Can be propagated from seed.

Uses: Flower petals give color to soups, custards, and rice; cookies; vinegars; crafts.

Caraway. *Carum carvi:*

grows twelve - twenty-four inches (30 – 60 cm) needs ten inches (25 cm) space when planting, needs sun. Can be propagated from seed.

Uses: Leaves in salads, teas, stews, and soups; seeds for flavoring cookies, breads, salads, and cheeses; roots can be cooked.

Chamomile, sweet false. *Matricaria recutita:*

grows one – two and half feet (30 – 75 cm) needs four – six inches (10 – 15 cm) space when planting, needs sun. Can be propagated from seed.

Uses: Tea, potpourris, garnish, crafts.

Chervil. *Anthriscus cerefolium:*

grows one – two and half feet (30 – 75 cm) needs fifteen inches (38 cm) space when planting, needs sun/partial shade. Sow seeds in early spring; needs light to germinate; does not transplant well, not heat tolerant.

Uses: Leaves in salads, soups, and sauces; teas; butters

A Basic Guide to Growing Herbs

Coriander (cilantro). *Coriandrum sativum:* grows twenty-four - thirty-six inches (60 – 90 cm) needs twelve – eighteen inches (30 – 45 cm) space when planting, needs sun/partial shade. Can be propagated from seed, goes to seed quickly so plant frequently.

Uses: Entire plant is edible; leaves in stews and sauces; stems flavor soups and beans; seeds in sauces and meat dishes, potpourris, and sachets.

Dill. *Anethum graveolens:*
grows three – five feet (90 – 152 cm) needs three – twelve inches (7 – 30 cm) space when planting, needs sun/partial shade. Can be propagated from seed, sow seed early spring.

Uses: Teas; seasoning for butter, cakes, bread, vinegars, soups, pickles, salads, etc.; flowers in crafts.

Nasturtium. *Tropaeolum* **spp**.:
grows fifteen inches (75 cm) needs six inches (15 cm) space when planting, needs sun. Can be propagated from seed, does not transplant well.

Uses: Leaves, stems, and flowers have a peppery taste; use in salads.

Parsley. *Petroselinum crispum:* grows six – eighteen inches (15 – 45 cm) needs six inches (30 cm) space when planting, needs sun. Can be propagated from seed, sow seed early spring; slow to germinate; soak in warm water; is a biennial grown as an annual.

Uses: Garnish; flavoring for salads, stews, soups, sauces, and salad dressings.

Perilla. *Perilla frutescens*: grows thirty-six inches (90 cm) needs three – six inches (7 – 15 cm) space when planting, needs sun. Can be propagated from seed,

Uses: Decorative plant; flavoring oriental dishes.

Summer savory. *Satureja hortensis:*
grows twelve – eighteen inches (30 – 45 cm) needs ten – twelve inches (25 – 30 cm) space when planting, needs sun. Can be propagated from seed, sow seed in early spring, cuttings

Uses: Mild peppery taste; used with meat, cabbage, rice, and bean dishes, stuffing, teas, butters, and vinegars.

BIENNIAL AND PERENNIAL HERBS.

Angelica. *Angelica archangelica:*
grows two – three feet (60 – 90 cm) needs three feet (60 cm) space when planting, needs partial shade. Can be propagated from seed,

Uses: Stems raw or in salads; leaves in soups and stews; teas; crafts; closely resembles poisonous water hemlock.

Anise hyssop. *Agastache foeniculum:*
grows three – five feet (90 – 152 cm) needs twelve - twenty-four inches (30 – 60 cm) space when planting, needs sun, light shade. Can be propagated from seed or division,

Uses: Attracts bees; edible flowers; leaves for flavoring or teas; crafts; seeds used in cookies, cakes, and muffins.

Artemisia. *Artemisia* spp.: grows two – three feet (60 – 90 cm) needs twenty-four inches (60 cm) space when planting, needs sun, partial shade. Can be propagated from division,

Uses: Wreaths and other crafts; aromatic foliage

Bee balm. *Monarda didyma:*

grows two – three feet (60 – 90 cm) needs twelve – fifteen inches (30 – 38 cm) space when planting, needs sun, partial shade. Can be propagated from seed or division, invasive rhizomes.

Uses: Attracts bees, butterflies, and hummingbirds; teas; flavors jellies, soups, stews, and fruit salads; edible flowers; dried flowers in crafts

Burnet, salad. *Poterium sanguisorba:*

grows twelve inches (30 cm) needs eighteen - twenty-four inches (45 – 60 cm) space when planting, needs sun, well-drained soil. Can be propagated from seed or division,

Uses: Cucumber-flavored leaves used in salads, vinegar, butter, cottage cheese, and cream cheese; garnish.

Clary sage. *Salvia sclarea:*

grows five feet (152 cm) needs twenty-four inches (60 cm) space when planting, needs sun. Can be propagated from seed, biennial,

Uses: Leaves in omelets, fritters, and stews; flavoring of beers and wines; oil.

Chamomile. *Chamaemelum nobile:*

two – eight inches (5 – 20 cm) needs eighteen inches (45 cm) space when planting, needs sun, partial shade; well-drained soil. Can be propagated from seed, stem cuttings,

Uses: Dried flowers for tea; potpourris, herb pillows.

A Basic Guide to Growing Herbs

Chives. *Allium schoenoprasum:* twelve inches (30 cm) needs twelve inches (30 cm) space when planting, needs sun, partial shade. Can be propagated from seed, or division,

Uses: Edible flowers; leaves for flavoring, eggs, soups, salads, butter, cheese, dips, spreads, etc.

Comfrey. *Symphythum officinale:*

three – five feet (90 – 152 cm) needs three feet (90 cm) space when planting, needs sun. Can be propagated from seed, cuttings, root division.

Uses: Safety of ingestion is highly questionable. Large, rambling plant; dyes, cosmetics.

Costmary. *Chrysanthemum balsamita:*

two – four feet (60 – 120 cm) needs twelve inches (30 cm) space when planting, needs sun, light shade. Can be propagated from division.

Uses: Garnish; fragrance.

Echinacea. *Echinacea angustifolia:*

one – two feet (30 – 60 cm) needs eighteen inches (45 cm) space when planting, needs sun. Can be propagated from seed or crown division. Uses: Entire plant edible; seeds in sausage and baked goods; leaves used with fish, vegetables, cheese spreads, and soups.

Fennel. *Foeniculum vulgare:*

four – five feet (120 – 152 cm) needs four – twelve inches (10 – 30 cm) space when planting, needs sun. Can be propagated from seed difficult to transplant.

Uses: Entire plant edible; seeds in sausage and baked goods; leaves used with fish, vegetables, cheese spreads, and soups.

Feverfew. *Tanacetum parthenium:*
two – three feet (60 – 90 cm) needs twelve inches (30 cm) space when planting, needs sun, partial shade. Can be propagated from seed or division.
Uses: Tea, crafts, dyes.

Geranium, scented. *Pelargonium* **spp**.:
twelve - twenty-four inches (30 – 60 cm) needs twelve - twenty-four inches (30 – 60 cm) space when planting, needs sun. Can be propagated from stem cuttings.
Uses: Teas, potpourris, sachets, jelly, vinegar, desserts.

Germander. *Teucrium chamaedrys:*
ten – twelve inches (25 – 30 cm) needs eight – ten inches (20 – 25 cm) space when planting, needs sun, partial shade. Slow to germinate from seed.
Uses: Attracts bees, decorative plant

Horehound. *Marrubium vulgare:*
twenty-four inches (60 cm) needs fifteen inches (38 cm) space when planting, needs full sun. Can be propagated from seed, cuttings or division.
Uses: Attracts bees; tea; flavoring in candy, crafts.

Hyssop. *Hyssopus officinalis:*
twenty-four inches (60 cm) needs fifteen inches (38 cm) space when planting, needs sun. Can be propagated from seed, stem cuttings or division.
Uses: Attracts bees and butterflies; mostly decorative usage, potpourris.

Lavender. *Lavandula angustifolia:* twenty-four – thirty-six inches (60 – 90 cm) needs eighteen inches (45 cm) space when planting, needs sun. Can be propagated from seed, stem cuttings.

Uses: Potpourris; herb pillows; crafts, vinegars and jellies.

Lemon balm. *Melissa officinalis:*

three feet (36 cm) needs twenty to twenty-four inches (50 – 60 cm) space when planting, needs sun, light shade. Can be propagated from seed, stem cuttings or division.

Uses: Teas; flavors soups, stew, fish, poultry, vegetables, and meat dishes; garnish; potpourris.

Lemon verbena. *Aloysia triphylla:*

two – five feet (60 – 152 cm) needs twelve - twenty-four inches (30 – 60 cm) space when planting, needs sun. Can be propagated from stem cuttings

Uses: Potpourris; herb pillows; lemon flavoring for drinks, salads, and jellies; teas.

Lovage. *Levisticum officinale:*

three – five feet (90 – 152 cm) needs two feet (60 cm) space when planting, needs sun, partial shade. Can be propagated from seeds, sow seeds late summer; division.

Uses: Seeds in breads, butters, and cakes; teas; leaves in soup, stew, cheese, cookies, and chicken dishes; root edible.

Marjoram. *Majorana hortensis:*

one – two feet (30 – 60 cm) needs twelve inches (30 cm) space when planting, needs sun, partial shade. Can be propagated from Stem cuttings, division, or seed

Uses: Flavoring for meats, salads, omelets, vinegars; jellies; teas; flower head for crafts.

A Basic Guide to Growing Herbs

Oregano. *Origanum vulgare* and *O. vulgare* subsp. *hirtum*:

twenty-four inches (60 cm) needs eight – twelve inches (20 – 30 cm) space when planting, needs sun. Can be propagated from cuttings, division.

Uses: Flavoring for tomato dishes, vegetables and sauces, etc.

Peppermint. *Mentha* x *piperita*:

thirty-six inches (90 cm) needs eighteen inches (45 cm) space when planting, needs sun, light shade. Can be propagated from cuttings and division recommended; invasive rhizomes.

Uses: Teas, fragrance.

Rosemary. *Rosemarinus officinalis*:

three – six feet (90 – 182 cm) needs twelve inches (30 cm) space when planting, needs sun. Seeds slow to germinate; use stem cuttings, layering, or division.

Uses: Teas; flavoring for vinegar, jam, bread, butters, stuffing, vegetables, stew, and meat dishes.

Rue. *Ruta graveolens*:

three feet (90 cm) needs twelve – eighteen (30 – 45 cm) space when planting, needs sun. Can be propagated from seeds, stem cuttings and division.

Uses: Decorative plant.

Sage. *Salvia officinalis*:

eighteen – thirty inches (30 – 75 cm) needs twelve inches (30 cm) space when planting, needs sun. Can be propagated from seeds (grows slowly), stem cuttings and division layering.

Uses: Seasoning for vegetable and egg dishes; stuffings.

Sage, pineapple. *Salvia elegans:* two – three feet (60 – 90 cm) needs twenty-four inches (60 cm) space when planting, needs sun. Can be propagated from stem cuttings

Uses: Attracts hummingbirds and butterflies; teas; potpourri; cream cheese; jams, jellies.

Santolina. *Santolina chamaecyparissus:* twenty-four inches (60 cm) needs two – three feet (60 – 90 cm) space when planting, needs sun, needs good drainage. Can be propagated seeds, Slow to germinate from seeds. Stem cuttings, layering, or division.

Uses: Dried arrangements and potpourris; accent plant.

Sorrel. *Rumex* **spp.**:
 three feet (90 cm) needs twelve inches (30 cm) space when planting, needs sun. Can be propagated from seed.

Uses: Flavoring of soups, butters, omelets; some species of sorrel are toxic.

Southernwood. *Artemisia abrotanum:*
four feet (120 cm) needs eighteen inches (45 cm) space when planting, needs sun, well drained soil. Can be propagated from stem cuttings, division.

Uses: Teas; sachets; potpourris.

Spearmint. *Mentha spicata:*
eighteen inches (45 cm) needs eighteen inches (45 cm) space when planting, needs sun, partial shade. Cuttings or division recommended; invasive rhizomes.

Uses: Teas; flavors sauces, jellies, and vinegars; leaves in fruit salad, peas, etc.

Sweet marjoram. *Origanum majorana:* eight inches (20 cm) needs twelve inches (30 cm) space when planting, needs sun. Can be propagated from seed, division or cuttings.

Uses: Flavors tomato sauces, eggs, etc. Leaves in salads, sauces, pizza, and meats.

Sweet rocket. *Hesperis matronalis:*

three feet (90 cm) needs twenty-four inches (60 cm) space when planting, needs sun. Can be propagated from seed,

Uses: Salads.

Sweet woodruff. *Galium odoratum:*

eight inches (20 cm) needs twelve inches (30 cm) space when planting, needs partial shade. Can be propagated from division,

Uses: Tea; sachets, dyes.

Tansy. *Tanacetum vulgare:*

three – four (90 - 121 cm) needs five inches (15 cm) space when planting, needs sun. Can be propagated from Seed or division

Uses: Toxic oil in leaves; decorative plant; crafts.

Tarragon. *Artemisia dracunculus:*

twenty-four inches (60 cm) needs twelve inches (30 cm) space when planting, needs sun. Can be propagated from Division or root cuttings, stem cuttings are slow to root.

Uses: Sauces, salads, soups, omelets, and vegetable, dishes.

Thyme, common. *Thymus vulgaris:*

four – twelve inches (10 – 30 cm) needs six – twelve inches (15 – 30 cm) space when planting, needs sun. Can be propagated from seeds, cuttings or division.

A Basic Guide to Growing Herbs

Uses: Teas; attracts bees; sachets; potpourris; flavoring for stews, soups, tomatoes, cheese, eggs, and rice.

Valerian. *Valeriana officinalis:*

two – five feet (60 – 150 cm) needs twelve - twenty-four inches (30 – 60 cm) space when planting, needs sun. Division is recommended over seeding.

Uses: Roots for flavoring; ornamental plant.

Yarrow. *Achillea millefolium:*

four feet (120 cm) needs twelve inches (30 cm) space when planting, needs sun. Can be propagated from seeds or division.

Uses: Crafts.

Winter savory. *Satureja Montana:*

twenty-four inches (60 cm) needs eighteen inches (45 cm) space when planting, needs sun. Grow in light, sandy soil from cuttings or seed; cut out dead wood.

Uses: Leaves used to flavor salads, soup, stew, and potpourris.

Wormwood. *Artemisia absinthium:*

thirty-six inches (90 cm) needs twelve inches (30 cm) space when planting, needs sun. Can be propagated from seed germinate slowly; use stem cuttings or division.

Uses: Bitter flavor; toxic if consumed in large quantity; ornamental plant, dried arrangements; insect repellent.

A Basic Guide to Growing Herbs

References

Coriander, http://www.theepicentre.com

Stinging nettle, https://www.alchemy-works.com/

How to Grow and Care For Calendula Flowers,
How to Grow Burdock,
How to grow chamomile
      www.gardenersnet.com

American Chemical Society Chamomile Tea: New Evidence Supports Health Benefits. *ScienceDaily*. Retrieved from http://www.sciencedaily.com

Add the romance of lavender to your garden, http://www.flower-gardening-made-easy.com

Lemon balm benefits
St. John's Wort Health Benefits and Information,
Echinacea Benefits and Side Effects
http://www.nutrasanus.com

Growing: Feverfew, http://www.thriftyfun.com

Three Tips for Successfully Growing a Culinary Herb Garden,

http://www.lawncare.net

Organic herb garden, http://www.planetnatural.com

Powdery mildew, http://gardening.about.com

http://herbgardens.about.com

Books

Hanson, Beth, **Designing an herb garden**, Brooklyn Botanic Gardens, New York City, NY.

Caduto, Michael J., ***Everyday Herbs in Spiritual Life,*** Skylight Paths Publishing, Woodstock, VT.

Castleman, Michael, ***The New Healing Herbs.***

www.ingramcontent.com/pod-product-compliance
Lightning Source LLC
Chambersburg PA
CBHW021955290426
44108CB00012B/1075